Study Guide

for

Wilson, Nathan, O'Leary, and Clark

ABNORMAL PSYCHOLOGY

INTEGRATING PERSPECTIVES

prepared by

Maureen A. Sullivan
and
Frank L. Collins, Jr.

Oklahoma State University

Allyn and Bacon
Boston London Toronto Sydney Tokyo Singapore

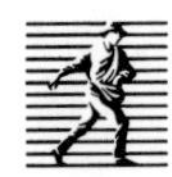

A Simon & Schuster Company
Needham Heights, Massachusetts 02194

ISBN 0-205-17583-X

Printed in the United States of America

10 9 8 7 6 5 4 3   01 00 99 98 97

Table of Contents

Preface

Chapter 1. Perspectives on Abnormal Behavior . . . 3

Chapter 2. Models of Abnormal Behavior. . . . 13

Chapter 3. Diagnosis and Clinical Assessment . . . 25

Chapter 4. Research Methods in the Study of Abnormal Behavior . . . 35

Chapter 5. Anxiety Disorders . . . 43

Chapter 6. Somatoform and Dissociative Disorders . . . 56

Chapter 7. Mood Disorders . . . 69

Chapter 8. Sexual Disorders . . . 83

Chapter 9. Substance-Related Disorders . . . 95

Chapter 10. Psychological Factors Affecting Health. . . .112

Chapter 11. Eating Disorders 123

Chapter 12. Personality Disorders 134

Chapter 13. Schizophrenia. . . .148

Chapter 14. Childhood Disorders. . . .164

Chapter 15. Mental Retardation and Autistic Disorders. . . .179

Chapter 16. Cognitive Disorders. . . .194

Chapter 17. Violence: Partner Abuse, Rape, and Child Abuse. . . .209

Chapter 18. Individual Psychological Therapies. . . .223

Chapter 19. Marital, Family, Group, and Community Therapies. . . .234

Chapter 20. Biological Therapies 243

Chapter 21. Legal and Ethical Issues. . . .253

Preface

This study guide is designed to help students who are using the second edition *of Abnormal Psychology: Integrating Perspectives* by Wilson, Nathan, O'Leary & Clark (1996). Each chapter has several components to help you learn the material from the text.

Each chapter is summarized, with the major headings, key terms and definitions, and important names underlined. This should not be used as a substitute for reading the chapter. It should help you identify the major points of the material presented; if this unclear, go back to the text and focus on the examples which illustrate specific points.

The Key Ideas and Objectives for Students highlights the major concepts and ideas in the chapter. They are phrased in the form of a question to help students determine whether they fully understand the material and to serve as a guide for testing yourself over the chapter in preparation for the exam.

The section on mental disorders in the movies is included so that you can choose a fun way to apply the principles and concepts of each chapter to popular media presentations of abnormal behavior and mental disorders. A brief summary of the movie, along with its illustration of specific symptoms, etiology, treatment, or issues, is presented. This is followed by specific questions to help the student apply his/her knowledge to the movie. These movies can serve as an interesting method for stimulating critical thinking, and they may help you to more easily remember these concepts and information.

For the chapters in which there is an accompanying case from Meyer and Osborne' (1996) *Case Studies in Abnormal Psychology,* one of the cases is selected. This case is then presented from the biopsychosocial perspective, which is a major perspective emphasized throughout the text. Studying these cases within this framework can serve as a review of the information on the etiology of each disorder. These can also serve as examples for the student in practicing viewing the remaining cases from the biopsychosocial perspective.

Lastly, sample multiple choice questions are presented to help students check their understanding of the material. These questions are taken from the text and are designed to sample major concepts from the chapter.

While much of the material presented in the text is quite detailed, this study guide can help students to select the most important information and to integrate the information into a conceptual framework. We hope that this study guide is helpful to many students.

CHAPTER 1 - PERSPECTIVES ON ABNORMAL BEHAVIOR

This chapter examines the concept of abnormal behavior from differing perspectives and explores the reasons for studying abnormal behavior. The prevalence and impact of mental health problems is presented in the context of recent epidemiological surveys. After reviewing the history of the field of abnormal behavior, an overview of the mental health professions is presented.

Why Study Abnormal Behavior?

Interest in identifying and understanding abnormal behavior is very common and is evident throughout history. Reasons for this interest range from self-awareness, to personal experience with a friend or relative who may have experienced difficulty. Many disorders are fairly common, such as psychosis, which is characterized by delusions (false beliefs) and hallucinations (false perceptions). The biopsychosocial perspective incorporates the interplay of biological factors (normal biology, disease processes, genetic influences), psychological factors (thoughts, feelings, and perceptions), and social and environmental factors.

What Is Abnormal Behavior?

It is difficult to determine what constitutes normal vs abnormal behavior. While some behaviors are distinctly different (e.g., psychotic behaviors) others are less clear. Judgments about abnormality depend upon standards for behavior which vary considerably across individuals and cultures. The Diagnostic and Statistical Manual of Mental Disorders (DSM-IV) incorporates a broad definition based on "painful symptom or impairment in one or more important areas of functioning."

Wakefield presents seven different views of abnormal behavior. Mental Disorder as Myth is based on Thomas Szasz's view that mental disorders do not truly exist, but were invented by psychiatrists to justify power and social control over others. Empirical evidence suggests that mental disorders do exist. Mental Disorder as Violation of Social Norms is based on the view that behaviors which are socially unacceptable are labeled as mental disorders. Homosexuality, which was once labeled a mental disorder in the DSM, is still considered a mental disorder by some. Mental Disorders as Whatever Professionals Treat is based on the assumption that professionals know how to identify and treat mental disorders. Mental Disorder as Statistical Deviance defines only those behaviors which are statistically deviant or rare as mental disorders. However, some behaviors associated with mental disorders may be quite common (e.g., suicide) and other rare behaviors or conditions (i.e., exceptional levels of intelligence) are not considered mental disorders. Mental Disorder as Biological Disadvantage defines mental disorders as those which interfere seriously with an individual's reproductive capacities. Mental Disorder as Unexpectable Distress or Disability views behavior that causes distress or disability or that is unexpected as mental disorders. However, distress resulting from poverty fits this definition but does not indicate mental disorder. Mental Disorder as Harmful Dysfunction incorporates two elements. What is harmful is a value based on social norms and the social context in which an individual functions. Dysfunction is a scientific term which refers to the failure of one's "mental mechanism" to perform the function for which it was designed. Wakefield considers this last definition as the best because it requires both scientific validation and consideration of social values.

Abnormal Behavior in the Contemporary United States

The prevalence of a disorder is the total number of people within a population with the disorder, while the incidence is the number of people within a population who have acquired the disorder within a specific time period. Epidemiological surveys examine a group to determine the incidence, prevalence and cause of disorders and may be used to determine the extent of mental disorders in the U.S. Three such surveys are reviewed.

The Midtown Manhattan Study surveyed mental health problems from 1952-1960 in New York City. The finding that almost 25% of those surveyed were emotionally impaired was both surprising and controversial. The higher rates of impairment in those of lower-class levels led to conclusions that racism and discrimination against the poor may substantially increase the risk of psychopathology.

The NIMH Epidemiologic Catchment Area (ECA) Study surveyed more than 20,000 persons in five U.S. cities and towns in the early 1980s and investigated the rates of specific mental disorders rather than general impairment. Based on regional differences in depression and drug abuse/dependence, it was concluded that the social environment affects both the rates and forms of psychopathology. Additional evidence that race and ethnicity play an important role in the development of psychopathology was obtained, which was consistent with the results of the Midtown Manhattan study. Approximately 1/3 of those surveyed met criteria for a specific diagnosis at some time during their lives; this supports the high rates of psychopathology in the U.S.

A national survey of depression in 8,098 persons from 1990-1992 also found evidence for significant psychopathology. Lifetime prevalence for major depression was 17%, with higher rates in women, young adults, and individuals with less than a college education. The biopsychosocial perspective has been used to explain and interpret these differences in prevalence. The Focus on Critical Thinking box (p. 12) asks students to consider potential differences between their own community and those used in the epidemiological surveys discussed.

Abnormal Behavior Through History

Abnormal behavior has been attributed to both natural forces, such as illness, and to supernatural forces, such as possession. While the prevailing explanation for mental disorders during the ancient world was based on supernatural forces, there were some exceptions. The Greek physician, Hippocrates, proposed that imbalances in the four essential fluids or humors led to most mental disorders. He also emphasized the role of stress, diet, heredity, and head injury in physical and mental problems and provided a detailed description of mental disorders such as mania, melancholia and paranoia. His views represent a naturalistic approach to understanding and treating mental disorders.

During the Middle Ages, views of mental disorder were influenced by the religious climate of the time and supernatural explanations of mental disorders predominated. Individuals displaying mental disorders were viewed as possessed by demons or as being punished for their sins. Exorcisms, food deprivation, or torture were the primary "treatments" for these persons. During the witch craze of the latter Middle Ages, those with mental disorders were tortured or killed because their difficulties were attributed to the devil.

The Renaissance period from the 15th to 17th centuries was characterized by a reaction against persecution of the mentally ill. Paracelsus proposed that the stars and the planets caused abnormal behavior, rather than demonic possession. Weyer argued that the mentally ill should not be held responsible for their actions and Scot argued that physical illness was the cause of mental disorders.

Asylums, or madhouses, were established during the mid-sixteenth century to house the mentally ill. The conditions at these facilities (chaining inhabitants, subjecting them to "mistreatments" and beatings) led to the reform movement which promoted humane treatment of the mentally ill. Those who were influential in this movement included Philippe Pinel in France, William Tuke in England, Benjamin Rush and Dorothea Dix in the United States.

The scientific study of the mentally ill developed from the asylums, which allowed for the systematic observation and study of large numbers of mentally ill. Pinel developed a classification system in which disorders were divided into the categories of melancholia, mania without delirium, mania with delirium, dementia and idiotism. Emil Kraepelin, a German physician working in the late nineteenth century, also developed a classification system for mental disorders. Using a scientific approach of systematic observation and description, he identified dementia praecox (later known as schizophrenia), and manic-depressive psychosis (now called bipolar affective disorder). He emphasized the role of the central nervous system and the brain in the development of mental disorders. Louis Pasteur's germ theory of disease was also influential in studying biological causes of mental disorders (e.g., syphilis).

The psychoanalytic theory was developed by Sigmund Freud at the end of the nineteenth century. Building from Jean-Martin Charcot's work with hysteria, and from the cathartic method or "talking cure" developed by Josef Breuer, Freud developed a theory that strongly influenced the field. The primary ideas were outlined in Freud and Breuer's Studies in Hysteria, published in 1895; these included the recognition of the effect of psychological factors on behavior, the superior efficacy of "talking treatments" over traditional harsh and moral treatments, the influence on behavior of thought patterns, impulses, and wishes of which the individual is unaware, and the need to study nonpsychotic behavioral disorders. Psychoanalytic theory dominated treatment of mental disorders until the mid-twentieth century and continues to influence the field today.

Adolf Meyer's psychobiology theory strongly influenced the field of psychiatry following World War I. He proposed that organic, psychological, and environmental factors contributed to psychopathology. This theory countered the emphasis that psychoanalytic theory placed on the primacy of unconscious factors in determining behavior.

These theories of etiology of mental illness are still influential today. However, the technological advances of neuroimaging, genetics, molecular biology and longitudinal research have provided important information regarding the etiology of disorders such as schizophrenia, bipolar affective disorder, and alcoholism. These developments should lead to more effective prevention and treatment in the future.

Treatment of psychiatric disorders has advanced considerably from the early treatments of bloodletting, special diets and other ineffective measures. Freud's talking therapies have been modified and continue to form the basis of much contemporary psychological treatment. Physical treatments have developed from early, largely ineffective treatments such as insulin coma therapy and psychosurgery, to more recent and effective drug therapy. Newly developed psychoactive drug treatments have proven helpful for such disorders as schizophrenia, bipolar affective disorder, and major depression and have contributed to the deinstitutionalization movement. Additional advances in the field of health psychology have contributed to the understanding and potential treatment of physical disorders such as cancer and heart disease.

The development of diagnosis and classification began in the U.S. and led to the Diagnostic and Statistical Manual of Mental Disorders (DSM). This system was designed to provide a uniform classification system and has been revised to reflect current theories and research.

Mental Health Professions

Clinical Psychology has traditionally focused on assessment of intelligence, personality, and psychopathology, and includes an increasing emphasis on research. Clinical psychologists receive intensive education consisting of a 4-year bachelor's degree in psychology or a related field, four to five years of doctoral academic work, plus a one-year clinical internship. Ph.D. programs provide extensive training in research and Psy.D. programs offer more extensive training in practice.

Psychiatrists are physicians who receive training in distinguishing between physical illnesses and psychopathology, and in psychopharmacology. Drug treatment for mental disorders has been the primary treatment provided by these professionals. Psychiatrists complete four years of college, four years of medical school, a year internship in a medical setting, and three or more years in a psychiatry residency.

Psychiatric social workers provide group therapy to families, couples, and other groups and often work in public settings. They help to provide resources such as financial and social support from community programs. Psychiatric social workers complete four years of college and two years at a university-based school of social work, and earn a master of social work degree.

Psychiatric nurses earn a B.S. degree and a diploma in nursing following a four-year nursing program. After completion of a licensing exam, most earn a master's degree in psychiatric nursing in a two-year program. Much of their work is in inpatient settings and is instrumental in providing a therapeutic milieu for patients.

KEY IDEAS AND OBJECTIVES FOR STUDENTS

After reading Chapter 1, you should be able to answer each of the following questions:

1. What factors are examined by the biopsychosocial perspective in abnormal behavior?

2. How is abnormal behavior defined from each of the following perspectives: standards of myth, social norm violation, what professionals treat, statistical deviance, biological disadvantage, unexpectable distress or disability, and harmful dysfunction?

3. What is determined by epidemiological surveys? According to these surveys, which groups have been found to have high rates of mental disorders?

4. What did early views of abnormal behavior stress? What do recent views focus on ?

5. Which persons were responsible for the reforms in mental health care?

6. Which publication outlines the current classification and diagnostic system used in the U.S.? Whose classification system is this based on?

7. When was Freud's psychoanalytic theory very influential in the field of abnormal behavior?

8. How has research on etiology, treatment, and diagnosis and classification affected knowledge in the last 20 years?

9. What are the mental health professions and how do the differ in training and provision of treatment?

Abnormal Behavior in the Movies

We have found that many students can relate to many of the issues critical to abnormal psychology through discussion of how abnormal psychology is presented in the popular media. In particular, students may want to rent and watch particular films that illustrate a specific disorder or concept relevant to the chapter and to discuss these issues in class. For each chapter, we have provided basic information on films that we find to be particularly useful with a summary of discussion topics and main points.

Two films illustrate the perspective that mental illness might be influenced by environmental factors.

1. <u>One Flew Over the Cuckoo's Nest</u> (1975, Republic Pictures Home Video, 133 min). This film provides a perspective from the view of a patient confined to a mental hospital for evaluation. Through the course of the movie, one begins to suspect that the staff are not necessarily more "sane" than the patients. In particular, the student may get the perspective that given certain life events, many people might develop abnormal behavior patterns. The film also highlights some of the less desirable aspects of institutionalization and could be useful in comparing differences in mental hospitals represented in this movie from contemporary treatment facilities.

2. <u>The King of Hearts</u> (1966, MGM/UA, 107 min). This is a French film with English subtitles. The movie begins near the end of World War I in a French town controlled by the Germans. The Allied Forces from Britain are advancing and the Germans decide to retreat. However, the German Commanders decide to rig a bomb to explode after they leave. The town's people realize what is happening and all abandon the town, leaving the residents of the local "Insane Asylum" as the sole residents. Word of this bomb gets back to the Britains who send in a soldier to disarm the bomb and secure the town. He ends up developing a relationship with those confined to the asylum. The film openly challenges the sanity of war when in the end the "insane" residents choose living in the asylum over being free to live with their "saviors." This movie should help you to consider the difficulty in defining abnormal behavior, and issues related to social norms and the cultural context.

Using Case Studies in Abnormal Behavior by Meyer and Osborne:
Concepts of Abnormality

Chapter 1 presents a brief overview of definitions of abnormality and presents the NIMH Epidemiological Survey to illustrate the prevalence of mental illness in the United States. The chapter then turns to examining the life and history of O. J. Simpson as an exercise to explore the issues of abnormality. The murders of Nicole Brown Simpson and Ronald Goldman which were allegedly committed by O. J. Simpson, are discussed in detail from the framework of the consistency or inconsistency in his behavior prior to the murders. The extent to which O. J. Simpson is diagnosable with any recognized mental disorder is explored. The author also presents a description of battered spouse syndrome and estranged spouse syndrome and fits these two patterns to Nicole Brown Simpson and O. J. Simpson, respectively.

A discussion of this case and the extent to which there is evidence of abnormality or mental illness can help students to apply the principles discussed in the first chapter.

Questions for the student:

1. Compare and contrast the definitions of abnormality as presented in the text to those presented in the case book. How are they similar? How are they different?

2. Can you think of other famous persons whose behavior may or may not be considered abnormal and/or diagnosable? Does the public use different definitions of abnormality or mental illness for the famous compared to the general public?

Sample Multiple-Choice Questions

1. Jim falsely believes that he is Jesus Christ. It is likely that Jim is suffering from a ______.
   a. hallucination
   b. dissociative identity disorder
   c. delusion
   d. narcissistic personality disorder

2. The fourth edition of the Diagnostic and Statistical Manual of Mental Disorders (DSM-IV) uses this definition: "a clinically significant behavioral or psychological syndrome or pattern ... associated with either a painful symptom or impairment in one or more important areas of functioning, " to define ______.
   a. insanity
   b. mental disorder
   c. psychosis
   d. neurosis

3. The ______ of a disorder is the total number of people within a given population who suffer from a disorder or condition.
   a. incidence
   b. disorder rate
   c. prevalence
   d. epidemiological rate

4. Tony believes that mental disorders can be caused by genetic factors, disease processes, and environmental and psychological factors. Tony believes that ______ forces cause mental disorders.
   a. natural
   b. supernatural
   c. external
   d. internal

5. ______ was known as "the father of American psychiatry."
   a. Sigmund Freud
   b. William Tuke
   c. Philipe Pinel
   d. Benjamin Rush

6. _______ is the most common psychosis and is characterized by hallucinations, delusions, profound problems in thinking, and bizarre behavior.
   a. Dementia
   b. Schizophrenia
   c. Delirium
   d. Mania

7. Your friend tells you about a technique that can be used to discover the emotional conflicts behind patients' problems. She explains that the technique is to have patients talk freely to the therapist and through this free association the emotional conflicts will eventually be revealed. You tell your friend that this is ______ technique.
   a. Jean-Martin Charcot's
   b. Sigmund Freud's
   c. Josef Breuer's
   d. Adolf Meyer's

8. Howard was given the medication Prozac in order to treat his depression. Howard is receiving ______ type of therapy.
   a. moral treatment therapy
   b. psychoanalytic therapy
   c. pharmacotherapy
   d. paratherapy

9. Persons who graduate with a Ph.D. or a Psy.D. and have a minimum of one year in a clinical internship are called ______.
   a. psychiatrists
   b. clinical psychologists
   c. psychiatric social workers
   d. psychiatric nurses

10. Chapter one of your casebook presented the case of O. J. Simpson. According to Meyer and Osborne, ______ is a term used to describe the behaviors which O. J. Simpson displayed.
   a. battered spouse syndrome
   b. estranged spouse syndrome
   c. battering spouse syndrome
   d. aggressive spouse syndrome

Answer Key

1. c
2. b
3. c
4. a
5. d
6. b
7. b
8. c
9. b
10. b

CHAPTER 2 MODELS OF ABNORMAL BEHAVIOR

Creating Models of Abnormal Behavior

Models are used to understand the development of mental disorders and to foster treatment and prevention. Early models focused on supernatural and natural influences, while more recent models emphasize social and psychological factors. The chapter presents six contemporary models of psychopathology, each of which focuses on biological, social and psychological factors. The biological model emphasizes disordered brain metabolism. The psychodynamic and humanistic models stress disturbed psychological processes. The social consequence model and the behavioral model focus on the reciprocal interaction of social and psychological factors. The biopsychosocial model studies the interactions of social, psychological and biological factors, and is emphasized throughout the text because of its comprehensiveness.

The Biological Model

This model assumes that the principal causes and most effective treatments are biological. It has been called the disease model because of its focus on symptoms; however, the biological model also incorporates factors such as genetics and brain injury, which are not linked to disease. This model has its roots in the ancient Greeks and Romans, and gained prominence during the seventeenth and eighteenth centuries. Emil Kraeplin's work on disease and the link to dementia praecox can be applied to the manic-depressive or bipolar disorders.

Three assumptions underlie the model. First, impairment or dysfunction of the brain causes mental disorder. Second, accurate diagnosis of mental disorders requires the identification of the impaired brain functioning. Third, treatment is directed towards modifying or eliminating the brain dysfunction. The cognitive disorders (delirium, dementia, and amnestic and other cognitive disorders), are serious brain disorders which can usually be diagnosed with new technological procedures. Technological advances such as neuroimaging, and molecular genetics have resulted in rapid advances in understanding of brain functioning and mental disorders, such as delirium, dementia, and amnestic disorders. Other disorders such as schizophrenia, mood disorders, and alcohol abuse/dependence have also been linked to brain dysfunction.

The biological bases of normal and abnormal behavior are examined by reviewing the nervous system, brain, and endocrine system and their functions. The nervous system is a complex system which affects thought, perceptions, and movements. It is composed of neurons, which are specialized cells which receive information from sensory receptors and which transmit messages to other neurons, to muscles and glands. Figure 2.1 on p. 31 of the text diagrams the parts of a neuron, including the dendrite which receives nerve impulses from other neurons, the axon which transmits nerve impulses to other neurons, and the synapse. Neurotransmitters are chemicals which carry nerve impulses, and norepinephrine, serotonin, and dopamine have been linked to symptoms of schizophrenia and mood disorders.

The nervous system is graphically presented in Figure 2.2 on p. 32 of the text. The central nervous system includes the brain and the spinal cord. The peripheral nervous system in composed of the somatic system (which controls skeletal muscles and voluntary movements of walking, talking, etc.), and the autonomic system (which influences heart, blood vessels, and other internal organs involved in physiological reactions of emotion). The autonomic system is composed of the parasympathetic division (which regulates normal bodily functions, such as heart rate and digestion), and the sympathetic division (which energizes or activates the organs in response to stress).

The brain can be divided into the hindbrain, the midbrain, and the forebrain. The hindbrain controls autonomic nervous system functioning. The midbrain contains the reticular activating system which is the "sleep-wake" center and also mediates attentional processes. The forebrain controls the ability to speak, think, plan and remember. It is composed of the thalamus and hypothalamus, which work in conjunction with parts of the cerebral cortex to mediate emotion, pain and pleasure, and aggression. The thalamus, hypothalamus, and parts of the cerebrum constitute the limbic system, which is responsible for the physical expression of emotion.

The cerebrum or cerebral cortex is involved in thinking, feeling, perceiving, and reflecting. Its sensory function involves receipt of information from the sense organs and processes it for later recall or immediate response. Its motor function controls movements of muscles. Its associational function links the parts of the cerebral cortex together, facilitating reasoning, planning, memory, creativity, and problem-solving. The cerebral cortex is divided into two hemispheres, each of which has four parts (see Figure 2.4 for a diagram). The temporal lobes control visual information processing, long-term memory, emotional experience, and sound recognition. The parietal lobes control touch recognition, and part of the left parietal lobe is involved in speech. The occipital lobes are involved in visual perception. The frontal lobes are involved in problem-solving, high-level reasoning, remembering, and social cognition. Structurally the two hemispheres appear identical, yet the functions and involvement in psychopathology are different for each. Both autism and schizophrenia have been associated with left hemisphere dysfunction.

The endocrine system includes the: pituitary gland, or master gland, which releases hormones and controls the other glands; the adrenal glands produce hormones such as cortisone and corticosterone, which regulate metabolism, and epinephrine and norepinephrine; and the gonadal glands which produce sex hormones. Prolonged stress interferes with endocrine system functioning.

Genetic factors in normal and abnormal behavior are studied by focusing on genes and chromosomes. Genes are the basic units of heredity and are arranged in a specific order along chromosomes. Most individuals have a unique genetic make-up. Fraternal or dizygotic twins result from separate fertilized ova. Identical or monozygotic twins, however, result from the same fertilized ova, and therefore, share the exact same genetic make-up, and are useful in studying the effects of heredity and environment on psychopathology.

A phenotype is an observable characteristic, such as height, hair color, and temperament and personality. A genotype refers to an array of genes which a person possesses, which is hereditary. Most traits are based upon multiple gene pairs. However, phenotypes are also affected by environmental factors. Meehl's stress-diathesis theory proposes that although some people inherit or develop predispositions (diatheses) to particular disorders, they will not emerge until or unless environmental stressors (death, divorce, disease, injury) are sufficient to convert the genetic predisposition into the actual disorder. This interactional model has been very influential in research on the etiology of mental disorders.

Behavioral genetics and gene-environment interactions are explored through specialized methodological designs. Family studies assume that heredity is a factor if the rate of a mental disorder is higher in the families of index cases or proband cases (affected patients) than in nonfamily members; however, the role of environment cannot be controlled with this design. Pedigree studies are similar in that distant relatives are examined for mental disorders to determine the extent to which the gene responsible for the disorder is dominant, recessive, or sex-linked. This can help to identify genetic "markers" which help locate the gene or genes responsible for the disorder.

Twin studies yield greater control over genetic and environmental factors since the genetic overlap among co-twins is known and environmental influences are thought to be the same for each twin. Evidence of heritability is found when the concordance rate is higher among monozygotic twins than among dizygotic twins. Schizophrenia, depression, alcoholism, and autism have been linked to genetics through twin studies. Adoption studies provide greater control over environment. Greater rates of alcoholism have been found among adoptees whose biological parents were alcoholic than among those whose adoptive parents were alcoholic. Similar findings have been reported for schizophrenia and for some personality traits.

Molecular genetics involves the search for the location of the gene or genes responsible for certain disorders. The chromosome and gene for Huntington's chorea have recently been isolated. Work is progressing with Alzheimer's disease, manic-depressive illness, and schizophrenia. These findings should lead to improved treatment and prevention of mental illness.

The biological model has reduced the stigma associated with mental illness and has led to more humane and effective treatments. It has also led to more scientific study of mental illness which has yielded improved diagnosis and treatment. However, this model cannot account for the role of other important factors, such as poverty and discrimination, and does not promote attention to society's role in the development of psychopathology. The text turns to the history of Malcolm X and applies the biological model.

The Psychodynamic Model

This model proposes that human behavior is strongly influenced by unconscious psychological processes of which we are largely unaware. Sigmund Freud's psychoanalytic theory is based on his structural theory of personality which is comprised of the id, ego, and superego. The id is the source of two basic, primitive drives and desires: the libido or life instinct involves primarily sexual drives; the thanatos or death instinct includes aggressive and destructive drives. The id operates on primary-process thinking, characterized by sexual fantasies, anger, jealousy, selfishness, and envy. The id is guided by the pleasure principle to maximize pleasure, and often conflicts with society's rules. The ego tempers and controls the id's primitive drives to conform to realistic demands of the environment. This involves secondary-process thinking, or reason and logic, in accordance with the reality principle, as the ego seeks to reduce conflict with society's rules. The ego, thus, acts as the executive manager of the personality. The superego is the earliest source of the conscience and possesses the ability to distinguish right from wrong. An overly restrictive superego could result from highly critical and punitive parenting, which would adversely affect later functioning.

Freud also proposed five stages of psychosexual development. The oral stage (birth-18 mos) is characterized by the involvement of the mouth, lips and tongue to satisfy the libido. During the anal stage (18 mos-3 yrs), pleasure is derived from anal and urinary sphincter muscles, and the newly developing control a child gains over his/her parents. In the phallic stage (3-6 yrs), pleasure is gained from the genitals and children must resolve strong conflicts with their parents. The Oedipus and Electra complexes occur during this stage, which involve sexual and aggressive feelings towards parents. The genital stage occurs with the onset of puberty and involves learning the pleasures and dangers of adult sexuality. The text again examines the life of Malcolm X, using the psychodynamic perspective.

Defense mechanisms are important processes whereby the ego deals with attack from the environment, the id, or the superego. Neurotic anxiety occurs when id impulses threaten to overcome the ego. Moral anxiety involves guilt and shame resulting from an overly harsh and punitive superego. Objective anxiety occurs when real danger is encountered. Table 2.1 on page 45 presents the major defense mechanisms and how they function.

Several of Freud's followers rejected the idea that infants and young children have unconscious sexual feelings towards their parents which could lead to psychopathology. Carl Jung focused on problems that the patient's parents experienced when they were a child. Alfred Adler emphasized the role of feelings of inferiority, while Otto Rank focused on the role of birth trauma and the development of psychopathology. The impact of culture and society and personality was emphasized by Karen Horney, Erich Fromm, and Erik Erikson. Horney attributed anxiety and depression to conflicts in three interpersonal areas: moving toward people, moving against people, and moving away from people. Erikson proposed an alternative, eight-stage model of development (p. 47). The ego psychologists, Heinz Hartmann, Rene Spitz, and Margaret Mahler, emphasized the importance of the ego and its defenses. Heinz Kohut's self-theory addressed the role of self-defects and the individual's view of him/herself in relation to others.

Psychoanalytic theory has highly influenced the study of mental illness and focused attention on the importance of childhood experiences. Freud demystified mental illness by constructing a comprehensive model. His focus on transference and countertransference, his in-depth clinical narratives, and his techniques significantly affected the practice of therapy. Criticism of his theory centers on the nonempirical basis for his theory and the difficulty in testing the theory. Additional criticisms involve the emphasis on abnormality, the limited applicability to prevention and early intervention, and questions about the degree to which the theory can be applied in an universal way.

The Humanistic Model

This model emphasizes unique human consciousness, the individual's perception of reality, and the uniqueness and worth of each individual. Each person is assumed to have the ability to grow emotionally and intellectually to realize his or her full potential. Carl Rogers proposed the person-centered theory of personality, which assumes that personality results from one's perceptions and interpretations of the world, as well as from biology and learning. The fourteen principles of his theory are summarized on page 50 of the text. Abraham Maslow described the process of self-actualization whereby each person achieves his/her unrealized potential, despite the inevitable frustrations of life. His hierarchy of needs is presented in Figure 2.6 on page 51. While the humanistic theory is more optimistic than the psychodynamic model, but is not a comprehensive model which can fully account for the development of mental illness.

The Behavioral Model

John B. Watson founded behaviorism as an objective branch of science with the goal of predicting and controlling behavior. The role of learning in the development of personality and psychopathology is critical, and learning occurs through classical conditioning, operant conditioning, and observational learning.

Classical conditioning occurs when an unconditioned stimulus (UCS) and a conditioned stimulus (CS) are repeatedly paired to produce a conditioned response (CR) which is similar to the unconditioned response (UCR). The unconditioned stimulus and unconditioned response are naturally occurring processes. The contiguity and contingency of the stimuli, as well as the value of the UCS and the relevance of the CS to the UCS can affect the speed and strength of the conditioning. Ivan Pavlov's research provided early empirical evidence of the role of classical conditioning in determining behavior. Through stimulus generalization (when a CR is linked to other stimuli which are similar to the CR) and higher-order conditioning (when a CS effectively becomes an UCS), complex associations can be formed.

Operant conditioning stemmed from Thorndike's law of effect, which states that behaviors associated with satisfying consequences are strengthened and thus more likely to be repeated, whereas those linked to unsatisfying consequences are weakened and less likely to be repeated. B. F. Skinner established the principles of operant conditioning and was very influential through his writing and his methodology of single-case designs. The discriminative stimulus refers to the information our environment provides us about the likelihood that our responses will be rewarded, ignored, or punished. The operant response refers to the voluntary responses which produce reinforcement or punishment. The reinforcing stimulus refers to the rewarding or punishing consequences of the operant response. When the reinforcing stimulus is rewarding, reinforcement occurs and the response is likely to be repeated. When the reinforcing stimulus is aversive, punishment occurs and the response is less likely to be repeated. These principles have had a significant impact, especially in designing therapeutic programs, especially in working with children who are aggressive, mentally retarded, or psychotic.

The behavioral model has fostered the emphasis on research and empirical data and has examined factors which are not addressed in the biological and psychodynamic models. The model has been criticized for deemphasizing the role of genetics and cognition.

Social Learning Theory stems from classical and operant conditioning, but focuses on observational learning, or modeling. This refers to a mode of learning in which one watches others engaging in various behaviors, but does not actually engaging in the behavior. Albert Bandura developed this model, which has been used extensively in the treatment of phobias. Self-control or self-regulation extends the model to explain the situation in which a person learns to control his/her behavior by choosing to pursue certain behavioral alternatives and by establishing rewards and punishments in accordance with one's own performance standards. Reciprocal determinism refers to the reciprocal interaction of behavior, cognitive factors, and environmental influences in learning and behavior. Self-efficacy refers to people's beliefs about their ability to exercise control over events that affect their lives. This model incorporates thoughts and feelings in learning and has been applied to interventions. The model has been criticized for the difficulty with which thoughts and feelings can be measured and for the neglect of genetic and biological factors.

Cognitive-behavioral approaches have heavily influenced treatment. The role of attributional processes (explanations we use to explain our successes and failures to ourselves) have been addressed in the therapy process as well. Treatment is based on teaching more adaptive ways to relate to the environment, such as problem-solving.

The Social Consequence Model

This model emphasizes the impact of belonging to certain groups in society on group members. Societal attitudes and behavior to persons based on their gender, ethnicity, race or SES are believed to affect their behavior and risk for psychopathology. Epidemiological survey data from the Midtown Manhattan Study and the NIMH ECA Study also support this model. A consistent finding from these and other studies is the link between the rate of certain disorders and gender; this may reflect, in part, differences in society's attitudes towards men and women. Race and ethnicity have also been identified as risk factors for psychopathology, perhaps as a result of the stressful living conditions which many minority groups face. Lewis proposed a culture of poverty that perpetuates stressful living conditions which promote physical and psychological illness. This model examines the development of psychopathology from a much broader context - society rather than the individual - and therefore addresses factors which are neglected in the biological, psychodynamic, humanistic, and behavioral models. However, it is difficult to determine the manner and extent of the impact of these factors on psychopathology. Also, it is possible that these effects are in the other direction (i.e., poverty results from psychopathology) and this model does not address this issue.

The Biopsychosocial Model

While the biological, behavioral, social learning, and social consequences models have more empirical support than the psychodynamic and humanistic models, none of them sufficiently explains the development of mental disorders. The biopsychosocial model is a comprehensive model which examines the interactive effects of genetic/biological and environmental factors. The text uses alcoholism to illustrate the utility of this model in explaining the complexity of this disorder. This perspective will be used throughout the text in examining abnormal behavior and the development, treatment, and prevention of mental illness.

KEY IDEAS AND OBJECTIVES FOR STUDENTS

After reading Chapter 2, you should be able to answer each of the following questions:

1. How are models used and when are they most useful?

2. What are the assumptions of the biological model?

3. What information regarding neurotransmitter excesses or deficits and the etiology of many mental disorders have been gathered in the last 20 years?

4. How have advances in behavioral and molecular genetics aided these investigations? How have neuroimaging techniques affected these investigations?

5. What are the assumptions of the psychodynamic model?

6. What are the components of Freud's structural theory of personality?

7. According to Freud, how do libidinous pleasure and different kinds of cognitive and psychological growth take place during each stage of psychosexual development?

8. How do the ego's defense mechanisms vary and how do they operate?

9. What are the assumptions of the humanistic model?

10. According to the behavioral model, what plays the key role in the development of behavior?

11. What are the three principal modes of learning that are crucial to acquiring new behavior and modifying existing behavior?

12. From what research area did social learning theory develop and what are its primary assumptions?

13. What are the assumptions of the social consequence model?

14. What are the components of the biopsychosocial model? How well does it explain normal and abnormal behavior?

Integrating Perspectives
A Biopsychosocial Model

Exploring the Biopsychosocial Perspective with Malcom X. Use the life of Malcolm X to demonstrate the biopsychosocial model and the interactive effects of biological, psychological, and social factors.

Biological Factors

•Genetic transmission of some or all of his parents' emotional distress: A fragile, intelligent, emotionally sensitive mother who developed a chronic psychosis; An abusive, violent, visionary father whose emotional instability was principally characterized by frequent ups and downs in mood.
•Malcolm clearly inherited his intelligence from both his parents.
•His father, a leader whose anger and inconsistency reduced the effectiveness of his leadership, could nonetheless have been a principal source of Malcolm's interpersonal and leadership skills.

Psychological Factors

•Malcolm's father was murdered and his mother began the slow process of mental disintegration when Malcolm was 6.
•Throughout his childhood, Malcolm experienced overwhelming stress from multiple environmental sources.

Social Factors

•At one time or another, as a child, Malcolm lived:
1) with an emotionally fragile, loving, highly stressed mother.
2) with an abusive and violent father who set very high standards for him.
3) with a supportive, loving group of seven siblings - until a state agency decided to break up the family following his mother's hospitalization.
4) in a difficult foster-family setting.
5) under the constant threat of violence.

The extent to which biological, psychological, and social factors contributed to the paradox that is Malcolm X - drug addict, alcoholic, intermittent depressive, petty criminal, and visionary leader of his people, is difficult to determine. But Malcolm X's life can be used as an illustration of the biopsychosocial model to help students tie together what they have read in the chapter.

Clinical scientists have for some time acknowledged the interactive role of biological, environmental, and social factors in understanding and treating psychopathology. Genetic transmission of some or all of his parents' emotional distress could have accounted in part for Malcolm's later substance-related disorders and depression. Although Malcolm didn't remember his childhood as having been so terrible, it does appear that way when one reads his autobiography.

Questions:

1. Imagine treating Malcolm X based on only one of the above factors. Which would you choose?

2. To what extent did the fact that his father was murdered and his mother deteriorate emotionally contribute to Malcolm's lifelong quest for emotional and physical autonomy and independence?

3. How likely is it that the multiple environmental stressors he experienced have the consequence of making Malcolm hypervigilant and suspicious as an adult?

Sample Multiple-Choice Questions

1. The ______ model of psychopathology emphasizes the role of disordered brain metabolism in determining the causes of mental illness.
   a. behavioral
   b. biopsychosocial
   c. biological
   d. humanistic

2. The two major divisions of the peripheral nervous system are the _____________ nervous systems.
   a. sympathetic and parasympathetic
   b. sympathetic and central
   c. autonomic and central
   d. autonomic and somatic

3. According to Freud, the _______ is the source of inherited, primitive drives, and is guided by ______ thinking.
   a. id, primary process
   b. ego, primary process
   c. id, secondary process
   d. ego, secondary process

4. Leo is two and one-half years old. He experiences sexual gratification through contracting and relaxing the sphincter muscles that control the elimination of bodily waste. According to Freud, he is in the ___________ stage.
   a. anal
   b. oral
   c. latency
   d. phallic

5. When Janet was a child, her parents were very punishing and were critical of all of her accomplishments. As she grew up, she developed a very punitive superego. Today, no matter how often people tell her what a wonderful mother she is, Janet always feels guilty for not being a better mother to her children. According to Freud, Janet is suffering from _____________ anxiety.
   a. neurotic
   b. moral
   c. objective
   d. all of the above

6. According to Maslow's theory, the needs of safety can be satisfied only after ______ are satisfied.
   a. self-actualization needs
   b. esteem needs
   c. needs to belong
   d. physiological needs

7. Gerry smells his mother's lasagna while he's eating a serving of it. The next time his mother cooks lasagna, Gerry's mouth waters as soon as he smells it, even though he hasn't tasted any yet. In this situation, the smell of the lasagna is the ____________.
   a. unconditioned stimulus
   b. conditioned stimulus
   c. unconditioned response
   d. conditioned response

8. Researchers who study society's biased attitudes and reactions towards minority groups and how they influence psychopathology would be exploring the _______ model.
   a. psychosocial
   b. psychobiological
   c. social consequence
   d. self-efficacy

9. Cloninger has applied the biopsychosocial model to explain alcoholism. He found that _______.
   a. all alcoholics are similar in family history of alcoholism, despite other differences among alcoholics
   b. all alcoholics are similar in signs and symptoms of alcoholism, but differ in other aspects of alcohol-related problems
   c. biological factors alone can account for differences in alcohol-related problems across alcoholics
   d. there are different patterns of interaction among biological, psychological and social factors among different alcoholics

10. The life of Malcolm X was characterized by a number of significant events which contributed to his psychopathology. _______ is an example of a biological factor.
    a. The support he gained from his siblings
    b. The murder of his father when Malcolm was 6 years old
    c. Living in a violent environment
    d. The chronic psychosis his mother experienced

Answer Key

1. c
2. d
3. a
4. a
5. b
6. d
7. b
8. c
9. d
10. d

CHAPTER 3 DIAGNOSIS AND CLINICAL ASSESSMENT

Diagnosis is the act of identifying and naming a disorder or disease by using a system of categorization. Clinical assessment is the process clinicians use to gather the information they need to diagnose, determine causes, plan treatment, and predict the future course of a disorder. The process of classification is based on an accurate assessment of past and present signs and symptoms. A sign is a characteristic feature of a disorder that may be recognized by the clinician, but not the patient. A symptom is a characteristic that the patient recognizes. The presence of signs and symptoms lead to classification or diagnosis. In abnormal psychology the most common classification system is the Diagnostic and Statistical Manual of Mental Disorders (DSM).

Chapter 3 provides an overview of the DSM classification system. In addition, three major categories of clinical assessment (Psychological Assessment, Assessment of Brain Disorders, and Behavioral Assessment) are used to illustrate how signs and symptoms of psychological disorders are measured.

The fourth edition of the Diagnostic and Statistical Manual of Mental Disorders (DSM-IV) has several improvements over previous versions of the DSM. First, operational criteria which outline and briefly describe the signs and symptoms considered in the diagnosis of each disorder have been modified and improved to better reflect substantial empirical, scientific findings. In addition, the DSM-IV reflects an increased reliance on empirical findings and is more sensitive to cultural differences in diagnosis than previous versions.

Consistent with previous versions of the DSM, DSM-IV requires a multiaxial diagnosis. The multiaxial diagnostic system divides abnormal behavior into two axes. Axis I is used to report all mental disorders except the personality disorders and mental retardation which are reported on Axis II. Axis III codes medical diseases or conditions and Axis IV codes psychosocial and environmental problems relevant to understanding or treating the mental disorders reported on Axes I and II. Axis V codes the Global Assessment of Functioning Scale used to assess the patient's overall level of functioning.

Three issues are important in evaluating the usefulness of any diagnostic system. These are (a) diagnostic reliability, (b) diagnostic validity, and (c) diagnostic bias. Diagnostic reliability refers to the extent with which clinicians agree on which signs and symptoms signal a specific disorder. The development of a common structure and an agreed upon set of signs and symptoms for each disorder (introduced in the third edition of the DSM) resulted in substantial improvements in diagnostic reliability of the operational criteria which continue to be used in the DSM-IV.

The capacity of a diagnostic system to identify and predict behavioral and psychiatric disorders accurately is known as diagnostic validity. A diagnostic system's ability to categorize current disorders accurately is termed concurrent validity; its capacity to predict future conditions is called predictive validity. Good diagnostic validity has been found for many of the DSM-IV disorders.

Psychological Assessment

Interviews are the most valuable tool used in psychological assessment. A diagnostic interview provides information on the patient's past and present behavior that have specific value for diagnosis. An assessment interview focuses on a wide range of topics, including assessment of personality, interpersonal behavior, and family functioning. An individual therapy interview brigs together the patient and therapist in an ongoing, extended relationship. Some interviews are highly structured and contain a detailed set of questions and always asked in the same order. Semi-structured interviews follow an outline but do not prescribe specific questions or require that the questions be in a particular order. The text presets an outline for a Mental Status Examination on page 79 which illustrates a Siam-structured interview.

Personality assessment attempts to measure enduring traits of character, skills, ability, and competence that makes on person different from another. Personality assessment methods are typically divided into projective methods and personality inventories. Projective tests ask respondents to impose their own structure and meaning on unstructured, ambiguous test stimuli. The Rorschach Inkblot Test consists of 10 inkblots, some black and white, some color, but all sufficiently ambiguous that so two viewers would see precisely the same thing. The goal of this test is to measure a person's projections (the meaning they give to the ambiguous inkblots) to gain insight into the unconscious determinants of behavior. The Thematic Apperception Test (TAT) consists of 31 stimulus cards that are shown, one at a time, with instructions to "tell as dramatic a story as possible" about each card. The TAT assumes that behaviors and feelings respondents attribute to the main character in a story represent their own tendencies and that respondents react to those aspects of the pictures that are most similar to important aspects of their own lives.

Other projective tests include sentence-completion tests that ask respondents to complete sentences beginning with such open-ended phrases as "My mother was..." or "The happiest time was ..." Another type of projective test asks people to draw familiar objects or people. The assumption behind projective drawings is that the content and form given to pictures provides uncensored information about their personality traits.

Personality inventories ask questions about respondents' behaviors, attitudes, experiences, and beliefs. Before publication, these inventories are evaluated by giving the inventories to a large number of people and analyzing the responses according to age, sex, socioeconomic status, diagnosis, and the like. This process is called standardization. General patterns are observed and established as what is considered normal for members of certain groups, called norms. The norms help the clinician to compare the responses of a patient with those of similar persons for a more accurate interpretation of the individual's personality.

One of the most widely used personality inventories is the Minnesota Multiphasic Personality Inventory (MMPI). This inventory asks respondents to answer "true" or "false" to a lengthy series of statements about themselves. The items used on the MMPI were initially selected because they differentiated among eight different diagnostic groups and nonpatient controls. The MMPI was modified in 1989. This revision, the MMPI-2, updated the language of some items and provided more contemporary norms for the restandardization. While the

MMPI-2 is considered more reliable than most projective measures of personality, many remain critical of the instrument because it relies on self-reports of behavior, thoughts, and feelings, which respondents can modify to suit their needs.

The Millon Clinical Multiaxial Inventory (MCMI) and its revision, the MCMI-II, are personality inventories designed specifically for diagnostic purposes. Their major emphasis is on the diagnosis of personality disorders, however, the MCMI-II has scales that parallel Axis I and Axis II diagnoses. The major criticism is that it underestimates the severity of depressive syndromes and overdiagnoses personality disorders.

The NEO Personality Inventory (NEO-PI) differs markedly from both the MMPI and MCMI in that the NEO is designed to study normal personality development, not for use with clinical populations. This scale provides measures of the "big five" personality traits: Extroversion, Agreeableness, Neuroticism, Conscientiousness, and Openness to Experience. These traits are called the "big five" because research has suggested that they explain a great deal of the variability in human behavior.

Intelligence Measures

The intelligence quotient (IQ) was an estimate of intelligence developed by Alfred Binet by calculating a mental age that represents performance on age-grouped tests and problems and dividing this by the child's chronological age and then multiplying this by 100. Thus a child who has an identical mental age and chronological age would have an IQ of 100. Higher scores indicate greater mental age compared to chronological age and lower scores indicate lower mental age. The scales originally developed by Binet are known today as the Stanford-Binet Scales and modified versions of these scales are commonly used for assessment of intelligence of children.

The Wechsler Adult Intelligence Scale-Revised (WAIS-R) is the revision of the first intelligence scale specifically developed for measuring intelligence in adults. This test evaluates eleven separate abilities, six verbal and five performance. Two other versions of the Wechsler scales have been developed. The Wechsler Intelligence Scale for Children-III (WISC-III) is designed for children between the ages of 5 and 16 and the Wechsler Preschool and Primary Scale of Intelligence (WPPSI) is for preschool children. All of these scales are based on the notion that intelligence is the sum of many separate abilities.

In recent years, experts have questioned the widely held notions of intelligence. Gardner developed a theory of multiple intelligences, which emphasizes the existence of several independent intelligences such as linguistic, logical-mathematical, musical, spatial, bodily kinesthetic, interpersonal, and intrapersonal. This model emphasizes that these different types of intelligences determine how successfully we interact with the world. Robert Sternberg developed the triarchic theory of human intelligence which stresses the role of intelligence in helping individuals adjust to new situations and environments. Both of these models require that we consider the cultural demands that the world placed on an individual's intelligence.

Assessment of Brain Disorders

Neuropsychological assessment of disordered brain function involves evaluating memory, problem-solving, and psychomotor tasks. The individual's performance on these tasks may reveal subtle brain damage before it begins to affect behavior. Two widely used assessment batteries are the Halstead-Reitan and the Luria-Nebraska Neuropsychologial Batteries.

Electroencephalography (EEG) is a technique for measuring the electrical activity of the brain. It involves placing electrodes on an individuals scalp. EEG waives can indicate brain injury or damage. For example, a normal, conscious, relaxed adult shows regular oscillating waves of between 8 and 12 cycles per sec called alpha waves. As the person becomes more excited, other patterns replace the alpha waves. For example, irregular, slow waves (less than 4 cycles per sec), known as delta waves, are typical of damaged or dying localized areas of the brain.

Before the early 1970s, radiological measures of the brain involved the use of a procedure called angiography in which a contrasting substance was injected into the bloodstream to show an outline of blood vessels in the brain visible on an X-ray. The development of computerized axial tomography (CAT) revolutionized brain imaging techniques by using computers to integrate multiple X-ray views of the brain to produce a single, reconstructed image. The computer can then look at a "slice," or cross-section of the brain and is sensitive enough to show the relationship among structures of the brain. This technology was the first to identify cortical atrophy, a reduction in brain volume which is characteristic of individuals with schizophrenia.

Magnetic resonance imaging (MRI) is a new techniques that may eventually replace the CAT as the preferred neuroimaging procedures. The MRI works by analyzing the nuclear magnetic movements of ordinary hydrogen in the body's water and fat. Not only is this imaging procedure more detailed, MRI does not expose subjects to radiation so repeated tests can be made without worry of overexposure. This procedure has allowed researchers to document brain abnormalities in individuals with schizophrenic, autistic, and bipolar disorders.

The X-ray, Cat scan, and MRI all provide precise representations of brain structure. Positron emission tomography (PET) permits direct measurement of information related to brain function by scanning receptors of gamma emissions from selected brain areas.

Behavioral Assessment

Behavioral assessment focuses on those specific aspects of a person's behavior that led the person to seek treatment. Detailed information is sought for (a) the target behavior, (b) antecedents, and (c) consequences. Target behaviors are the disturbed and disturbing behaviors as well as the thoughts and feelings that accompany them. Antecedents are the events and circumstances that typically precede the target behaviors. Consequences are the events and circumstances that typically follow the target behaviors.

Behavioral clinicians try, whenever possible, to observe their patients' troubled behaviors directly. However, usually, the best way to gather information about people is to ask them for it. One such method is the use of self-reports. Self-reports include the individuals accounts of the frequency of target behaviors, along with descriptions their antecedents and consequences. Some times this is obtained by having clients self-monitor thoughts and feelings using methods that ask the client to observe and record their own behavior over time.

Behavioral clinicians also rely on measures of bodily functioning, primarily autonomic nervous system (ANS) activity and muscle tension. Measures of overt behavior, subjective feelings and attitudes about the behavior, and the body's physiological responses are often compared to determine the extent with which these three systems are in agreement.

KEY IDEAS AND OBJECTIVES FOR STUDENTS

After reading the chapter, you should be able to answer each of the following questions:

1. What does diagnosis involve?

2. Upon what do mental health clinicians base their diagnoses?

3. How does the DSM-IV offer improvements diagnostic features? What are the primary components of this system and how do they affect diagnostic reliability and validity, sensitivity to individual differences, the possibility of diagnostic bias?

4. What are the different types of interviews?

5. What are the characteristics of projective tests and how do they supposedly reveal underlying personality traits?

6. What is the most commonly used objective measure of personality?

7. Who were the central figures in the history of intelligence testing?

8. What do the instruments used for neuropsychological assessment of disordered brain function involve?

9. What is electroencephalography (EEG) and what does it measure?

10. What are the two techniques most often used today to examine brain structure and how do they work?

11. What are the characteristics of behavioral assessment ?

12. How have behavioral clinicians developed assessment instruments?

13. How do behavioral clinicians rely on measures of bodily functioning to track therapeutic success, plan interventions, and sometimes actually intervene?

Sample Multiple-Choice Questions

1. __________ is the process used to gather information needed to identify, determine causes, plan treatment, and predict the course of a disorder.
   a. Assessment
   b. Diagnosis
   c. Intervention
   d. All of the above

2. Jack presents with frequent complaints of headaches, fatigue, chronic back pain, and lack of energy. These _____ may help his clinician identify which particular disorder Jack may have.
   a. signs
   b. symptoms
   c. syndromes
   d. behaviors

3. The current classification system used by most US mental health professionals today to assess abnormal behavior is the _____.
   a. DSM-II
   b. DSM-III
   c. DSM-III-R
   d. DSM-IV

4. Dr. T. is a psychologist who is interested in personality. Dr. T. believes that individuals reveal their underlying needs and conflicts to unstructured, ambiguous test stimuli. Dr. T. most likely uses what type of tests?
   a. Intelligence
   b. objective
   c. Projective
   d. Behavioral

5. Mary completed the MMPI-2 as part of a psychological assessment. Only one scale was highly elevated, while all others were within normal limits. This scale suggested that Mary has excessive concerns about her bodily functions and imagined illness. Which MMPI-2 scale is elevated?
   a. Schizophrenia
   b. Hypochondriasis
   c. Hysteria
   d. Paranoia

6. On the Binet scales, IQ is calculated by _____
   a. dividing mental age by chronological age, then multiplying by 100.
   b. dividing basal age by chronological age, then multiplying by 100.
   c. dividing developmental age by mental age, then multiplying by 100.
   d. diving mental age by basal age, then multiplying by 100.

7. Dr. G. always gives a WAIS-R as part of a neuropsychological evaluation. This allows Dr. G. to examine an individual's strengths and weaknesses, look at an individual's problem solving skills, and more. Which WAIS-R subtest would be the least likely to provide information regarding the existence of brain damage?
   a. Block Design
   b. Symbol Search
   c. Digit Span
   d. Digit Symbol

8. Electrical activity of the brain is measured by the _____.
   a. electroencephalograph
   b. electrocardiograph
   c. electromyograph
   d. PET scan

9. Diane's neurologist believes that Diane has a circulatory disease that is affecting her brain. Her physician wishes to use an imaging procedure designed to detect a substance injected into Diane's bloodstream. This procedure will enable her physician to view outlines of the blood vessels within the brain on an X-ray. Which procedure listed below best describes this technique?
   a. angiography
   b. PET
   c. CAT
   d. MRI

10. Andy is trying to stop smoking. His therapist has asked him to keep a detailed log of every cigarette he smokes. For each cigarette he smokes, Andy is to record the time of day, where he is (i.e., work, school, home, etc.), who else is around (alone, with friends, etc.), and the thoughts and feeling he has at that time. This technique is best described as _____.
   a. an objective assessment
   b. self-monitoring
   c. target behavior
   d. behavioral assessment

Answer Key

1. a
2. b
3. d
4. c
5. b
6. a
7. b
8. a
9. a
10. b

CHAPTER 4 RESEARCH METHODS IN THE STUDY OF ABNORMAL BEHAVIOR

The Scientific Study of Abnormal Behavior

Scientific study of abnormal behavior tries to discover patterns and trends which can be used as the foundation for general laws that explain apparently diverse bits of behavior. Reliability refers to the consistency of results obtained from a psychological measure. It can be established by consistency in the independent ratings of two different persons, or consistency in the ratings by the same observer at two different times. Validity refers to the accuracy of a test, or the extent to which the test measures what the test is intended to measure. Discriminant validity refers to a test's ability to accurately discriminate between those exhibiting the phenomenon (e.g., mental illness) from those who do not. Construct validity is established when a measure corresponds to other similar measures. Predictive validity refers to the ability of a test to predict the future course of a mental illness.

A scientific theory is an explicit and formal statement of a set of propositions designed to explain a particular phenomenon. A theory must meet three criteria: 1) it should clearly explain and integrate information currently known about the phenomenon in question; 2) it must be testable, using rigorous experiments designed to either support or refute it; and 3) it should stimulate research leading to new findings. Striegel-Moore's theory that eating disorders are the result of cultural norms for thinness is presented to illustrate the properties of theories. Theories can serve several purposes, such as providing an heuristic (stimulating new ideas and innovative research), and guiding therapists in clinical practice.

The benefits of research include the development of effective treatments (e.g., Prozac), establishing the truth about abnormal psychology and thereby disconfirming erroneous beliefs about the causes of mental illness.

Research Strategies

Controlled experiments randomly assign subjects to conditions and manipulate one variable (the independent variable) in order to measure its effects on another variable (the dependent variable). Operational definitions, or descriptions of constructs in objective, measurable terms, are necessary. The hypothesis is what an experiment is designed to test.

The internal validity of an experiment refers to the degree to which change in the dependent variable is due to manipulation of the independent variable. Alternative explanations must be ruled out. Spontaneous remissions and other factors which provide plausible explanations for changes in the dependent variable are confounds. Control groups are groups of subjects that are functionally the same as the experimental group on all dimensions except the one being manipulated, and can eliminate confounds. Random assignment is a procedure involving assigning subjects to groups so that each subject has an equal chance of being in either the experimental or control group; this improves the chances that subjects' characteristics will be equally distributed across treatment conditions in an experiment and cannot systematically influence the dependent variable. Figure 4.2 on page 111 presents the balanced placebo design used in research on alcohol effects and expectancy.

An alternative control strategy is the double-blind strategy in which both subjects and the researchers conducting the study are unaware of the manipulation. Studies of the effects of drugs on mental illness often use this design to limit the effects of expectancy.

External validity refers to the degree to which the findings of a particular experiment can be generalized to other subjects in other settings. Field research involves real-life settings and is designed to control for the potential artificiality of laboratory settings. It is difficult to conduct direct studies because of: the limits on conducting highly controlled studies in service-delivery settings, the difficulty in recruiting experienced therapists to participate, and finding sufficient numbers of patients with similar problems and characteristics to participate. Analogue research is an alternative which involves experimental treatment research conducted in the laboratory under highly controlled conditions with carefully selected subjects. This allows for standardization of treatment, and use of a wide range of subjective and objective measures of behavioral change. Homogeneous subjects with the same problem allow for the evaluation of the particular problem the treatment is best suited for. The more similar the analogue situation is to the natural or clinical situation, the greater the generalizability of results.

Quasi-Experimental methods are used when it is impossible to randomly assign subjects to experimental conditions. This method is useful to study pre-existing individual differences. One group consists of individuals with a known condition (e.g., an alcoholic parent) and the members of the other group will match the experimental group members on known personal characteristics that might confound the interpretation of results, but differ from the experimental group on the independent variable. Strong inferences about causation cannot be made with this design, however, because the two groups may differ on some unknown variable. In this instance, replication of results in subsequent studies can strengthen the confidence placed in the results of the first study.

Correlational designs assess the extent to which two or more variables are related. Information is gathered without altering subjects' experiences and therefore inferences about cause and effect cannot be made. A correlation coefficient is a number from -1 to +1 which describes the strength and direction of the relationship between two variables. "Three C's" can be used to help interpret a given correlation: one of the variables will be the cause, the consequence, or the correlate (related by virtue of a third variable) of the other.

Epidemiology is a correlational method that studies the prevalence, etiology and consequences of physical disease and mental disorders in a population. Epidemiological family studies investigate the interaction between genetic and environmental factors by measuring the rate of a disorder in the children of probands (those with the disorder). Longitudinal designs, which study one group of subjects repeatedly at different ages, can identify risk factors for developing a disorder. The case-control design involves matching a person with a clinical disorder with a control person who does not have the disorder but who is similar in age, race, sex, and socioeconomic status. Family aggregation evidence (findings in which the relatives of a person with a given disorder are more likely to have the disorder than would be expected by chance) do not control for environmental factors, however. Risk factors for disorders can also be identified from case-control studies.

Berkson's bias is a form of sampling bias in which people who have two or more medical or psychiatric problems are more likely to seek treatment than those who have only one problem; as a result, clinical samples are likely to contain more disturbed people than community samples. Epidemiological research, therefore, should be based on community samples in order to avoid erroneous conclusions.

Case studies examine a single individual through interviews, observations, and sometimes test scores, in order to better understand the individual. They are useful for describing the person's problem, relating it to present and past functioning, and forming hypotheses about the causes of the problem. Scientific benefit is derived when hypotheses are generated for testing in empirical studies. Clinical benefit is gained from the reporting and description of clinical methods applied to particular clients, but only when three criteria are met: 1) sufficient detail and precision in description of treatment methods to allow replication; 2) methods must be applied to specific problems; and 3) relevant personal characteristics of the patient are reported. Disadvantages include the inability to determine causality or efficacy of treatments.

Evaluating the Effects of Treatment

Single-case experimental designs were developed by B. F. Skinner to conduct controlled research and treatment with a single individual. Reversal designs are characterized by a baseline observation (A), a treatment phase (B), and a second baseline phase (A). If treatment is effective, then there should be a distinct improvement in phase B, but a return to previous levels in the second A phase. There are ethical and practical problems associated with returning an individual to baseline levels of functioning after an effective treatment; treatments may also not be reversible if permanent changes result from treatment (i.e., learning of new skills). Multiple baseline designs measure several responses to provide a baseline to evaluate changes against; each response is successively modified. If changes in a response only occur following intervention for that response, then a cause-effect relationship has been demonstrated. Generalization of treatment effects to multiple responses, however, can be problematic with this design. Advantages of single-case studies include: continual assessment over time to facilitates treatment modifications; results are replicated with the same subject over time which allows objective evaluation of treatment of problems not conducive to group methodology. Disadvantages include: possible interactions of subject variables with specific treatment techniques cannot be studied; generalization of findings beyond the individual is difficult.

Randomized group designs provide greater generalizability of findings. Waiting-list control groups are control groups in which patients are promised therapy after a period of time during which the experimental group receives treatment. The comparative outcome study, in which two or more specific treatments are compared with each other, is the best method for evaluating treatment efficacy.

Ethics in Psychological Research

Strict guidelines exist to protect those participating in research projects. Informed consent is the authorization granted by research subjects based on their understanding of what is involved in the research, and all aspects that may affect subjects' willingness to participate must be explained. Debriefing occurs after participation and provides a full account of the purpose of the study and any deception that was used. Institutional review boards at universities and medical schools ensure that ethical standards are followed. Ethical dilemmas, however, do still occur.

KEY IDEAS AND OBJECTIVES FOR STUDENTS

After reading the chapter, you should be able to answer each of the following questions:

1. What criteria must diagnosis meet in order to meet standards of scientific inquiry?

2. What are the requirements of reliability?

3. What is the definition of validity?

4. What is a scientific theory and what are its requirements?

5. How has scientific research contributed to our understanding of abnormal psychology?,

6. Why are controlled experimental methods necessary?

7. What is an independent variable and what is a dependent variable?

8. What are hypotheses?

9. What are the characteristics of an experiment that is internally valid and what does this mean?

10. What is a control group and how is it used?,

11. What is external validity?

12. What does random assignment ensure and why is it used?

13. What are quasi-experimental designs and when are they used?

14. What are correlational designs? What do they assess and what are their limitations? What does the correlation coefficient indicates?

15. How does epidemiological research use correlational methods and what is examined?

16. What are the characteristics and limitations of case studies? How do they differ from experimental methods?

17. What are single-case experimental designs and how do they differ from case studies?

18. What are randomized control designs and how can they be used?

19. What is the National Institutes of Mental health (NIMH), and what is its purpose?

20. What guidelines must be used with all research subjects?

21. How can the risks and benefits of clinical research be handled?

Sample Multiple-Choice Questions

1. Which of the following statements about the scientific study of abnormal behavior is FALSE?
   a. Its goal is to discover patterns of behavior to formulate general laws of behavior.
   b. It requires consistent and replicable diagnosis.
   c. It requires accurate measurement.
   d. It requires reliability but not validity.

2. Dr. Zhivago is developing a new measure for detecting depression in clinic patients. To ensure validity, she compared her measure with several other depression inventories. This will help establish ________ validity.
   a. discriminant
   b. construct
   c. convergent
   d. predictive

3. The belief that childhood autism was largely caused by cold, inexpressive parents who did not provide their children with the affection required is an example of a(n) ________.
   a. hypothesis
   b. myth
   c. theory
   d. risk factor

4. Jane hypothesizes that grade performance influences a student's mood. During her experiment she administered an easy task to all her subjects. However, she gave one group of subjects positive feedback and one group of subjects negative feedback (regardless of their actual performance), and measured their emotional response. In this study ________ is the independent variable.
   a. emotional state
   b. performance on the test
   c. easy task
   d. positive and negative feedback

5. Which of the following increases internal validity?
   a. Spontaneous remission
   b. Control groups
   c. Confounds
   d. Repeated trials

6. Scientists control for subjects' expectations in research by using ________.
   a. placebos
   b. independent variables
   c. dependent variables
   d. selection factors

7. There is a good chance that we will find a _______ correlation between time spent watching TV and grades in school.
   a. zero
   b. negative
   c. positive
   d. weak

8. Dr. Jones is interested in the effect divorce may have on children. He interviews adult subjects who report divorce when they were between 8 and 12 years old. He asks the same questions in a standardized way to allow for comparisons between subjects. He is using a ________.
   a. clinical survey
   b. structured interview
   c. structured assessment
   d. case study

9. A therapist engages in ten years of therapy with a patient diagnosed as having dissociative identity disorder (multiple personality disorder). When the therapy has concluded, the therapist uses her extensive notes, drawn from the ten years of clinical interviews with the patient. This history is then published so that others can learn from the therapist's experiences with her patient. This technique is known as a(n) ________ study.
   a. analogue
   b. epidemiological
   c. case
   d. naturalistic observation

10. Dr. Smith works in a hospital setting with people who have chronic schizophrenia. He is developing a treatment program to teach social skills to those getting ready to leave the unit and move to a group home. He wants to know if the social skills program is more effective than routine hospital therapy. He should use a ________ design.
   a. waiting-list control
   b. comparative outcome
   c. no-treatment control
   d. correlational

Answer Key

1. d
2. b
3. b
4. d
5. b
6. a
7. b
8. b
9. c
10. b

CHAPTER 5 ANXIETY DISORDERS

Anxiety disorders are the most common type of psychiatric disorder affecting people in the United States. Modern biological models trace the origin of anxiety to the brain. Biological models of anxiety have focused on sophisticated measures of brain functioning such as PET scans (See Chapter 3 for more discussion of PET scans) which can identify which areas of the brain are more active during anxiety states. Brain cells linked to anxiety are located in the portion of the brain stem known as the locus ceruleus. Electrical stimulation of these cells triggers fear, whereas destroying them inhibits fear. These cells have specific receptors for benzodiazepines, which reduce anxiety.

Anxiety plays a critical role in the Psychodynamic Model of Sigmund Freud. This model focuses on a painful tensions present in individuals that they seek to reduce. This anxiety is called neurotic anxiety and can be traced to early childhood conflicts. Reduction of neurotic anxiety comes about through the use of defense mechanisms. The most fundamental defense mechanism is repression which allows the ego to exclude threatening impulses from conscious awareness. This model has a strong historical influence on the study of anxiety disorders. Before the introduction of the third edition of the DSM, anxiety disorders were one of several disorders known as neurotic disorders or neuroses. Based on the psychodynamic model, each of these disorders was seen as a symbolic representation of intrapsychic conflict between the id and ego or the ego and superego.

David Barlow's biopsychosocial model of anxiety draws not only on cognitive and behavioral research but also on the psychology of emotion. He distinguishes between fear (a primitive, basic emotion that occurs automatically when we are threatened with real or perceived danger) and anxiety (a blend of different emotions, including anger, excitement, and fear itself). This model of anxiety suggests that due to heredity, some individuals have a biological vulnerability to stress and exposure to stressful life events activiates this vulnerability. Other individuals also have a psychological vulnerability to stress. Stress for these individuals is seen as unpredictable or uncontrollable. Individuals with both a biological and psychological vulnerability to stress develop anxiety disorders.

Social factors play an important role in the development of anxiety disorders, particularly with respect to gender issues. The "Thinking about Social Issues" focus box on page 136 provides an indept analysis of this issue with respect to agoraphobia which has a 3-1 ratio of women to men. Social factors which allow women to avoid difficult situations more easily than men is proposed as a possible explanation for this gender difference.

The distinction between fear and anxiety helps explain the differences between panic and anxiety. A panic attack is a sudden feeling of intense fear accompanied by various physiological symptoms. Thus, panic is the clinical manifestation of fear. However, rather than being a true emotional alarm triggered by real danger, panic is a false alarm because the danger is only perceived. Panic differs from anxiety in two ways: (1) in the specific thoughts associated with the anxiety and (2) in physiological responsiveness. Patients who experience panic report more thoughts about illness, dying, and collapsing than patients with other anxiety disorders.

Panic Disorder

The DSM-IV distinguishes between panic disorder with and without agoraphogia. Panic disorder with agoraphobia is diagnosed if the patient meets the criteria for agoraphobia in addition to those for panic disorder. The two most promising and influential theories of panic disorder are the biological model and the cognitive-behavioral model.

According to the biological model, panic is an unlearned alarm reaction, activated by a biochemical dysfunction, whereas other forms of anxiety are learned. Evidence supports this model. First, a genetic basis exists for panic disorder that seems independent of other anxiety disorders. Familial transmission of panic disorder appears to be genetically influenced. Second, panic disorder patients differ physiologically from normal people. Sodium lactate infusion produces panic in panic patients, but not normal controls. Third, PET scans show differences in brain function during sodium lactate infusions for panic patients and normal control.

The cognitive-behavioral model suggests that panic disorder results from the individual's catastrophic misinterpretation of normal bodily sensations. This catastrophic thinking is what Barlow sees as a psychological vulnerability.

Pharmacological therapy for anxiety disorders include antidepressant drugs such as Imipramine and Xanax, a high-potency benzodiazepine. The effectiveness of Xanax is unclear and a majority of patients who use Xanax become physically dependent. In general, drug therapies are less effective than psychological treatment.

Cognitive-behavioral therapies is an effective psychological treatment which focuses on teaching clients to reinterpret catastrophic thoughts so that they no longer trigger panic. Recent studies have found that a combination of cognitive-behavioral therapy and imipramine was more effective in the treatment of panic disorder than either pharmacological or psychological treatment alone.

Agoraphobia

While agoraphobia is typically associated with panic disorder, DSM-IV includes the diagnosis of Agoraphobia without a history of Panic Disorder. While this disorder is uncommon, far more women are affected than men. Most of the research on agoraphobia comes from the study of agoraphobics who had panic attacks. Agoraphobia, like panic disorder, appears to have a strong familial transmission. Other family factors that may play a role include pathological marriages wherein the wife uses her disorder as a way of controlling her husband or a husband might unconsciously encourage his wife in the dependency and limited social functioning as a way of controlling her. Cognitive-behavioral models suggest that once the initial panic or anxiety attack has occurred, the person increasingly avoids the original and related situations.

The most effective treatment of agoraphobia is the cognitive-behavioral therapy technique known as exposure treatment. Patients are encouraged to systematically and gradually confront the situations they fear and avoid. A combination of exposure treatment and imipramine has produced better results than either the drug alone or exposure treatment plus a drug placebo.

Specific Phobias

Specific phobia is an excessive fear of a specific object or situation. The opening case of Chapter 5 illustrates a case of claustrophobia, a type of simple phobia. According to biological models feel that heredity and genetics influence the development of simple phobias. The preparedness hypothesis predicts that our evolutionary past has prepared us to be afraid of objects or situations that, at one time, were associated with danger. This model has been used to explain why some fears, like fears of snakes or blood, are more common than fears of houses or flowers.

The psychodynamic model views phobias as transformed, unconscious neurotic anxiety. In other words, some deep-seated conflict is expressed as an irrational fear without our awareness.

The cognitive-behavioral model views phobias as primarily the result of classical conditioning wherein an object or situation is paired with a traumatic event. Observing some other person behaving fearfully is another way to acquire phobic anxiety. Two specific factors seem to be important in predicting when conditioning will lead to the development of a phobia. The first, controllability, refers to real or perceived ability to control or influence potentially threatening events. High levels of perceived control is called self-efficacy. Self-efficacy is a product of what we've learned we can and cannot handle. The greater our feelings of self-efficacy, the less vulnerable we are to developing phobic reactions in response to traumatic experiences.

Behavior therapy is an effective treatment for specific phobias. The most powerful method is exposure treatment, in which patients confront their phobic situations in a gradual and planned manner. Exposure treatments appear to work because they increase patients' self-efficacy. Individuals come to believe that they can cope successfully with the phobic object or situation.

Social Phobias

People with social phobias dread a variety of social situations because they fear being humiliated or embarrassed. There is debate as to whether or not social phobia is merely an extreme end of shyness or qualitatively different. Social phobias appear to be cross cultural, although different cultures express phobic problems in different ways. For example, the "Thinking about Multicultural Issues" example on page 148 discusses a Chinese disorder, Koro, a fear that the sexual organs will retract into the body, resulting in death. Likewise, the disorder, Taijin kyofusho (TKS) is defined as anxiety about offending others by blushing, emitting offensive odors or being flatulent, staring inappropriately, presenting improper facial expressions, or having physical deformities. Individuals with TKS are quire similar to the DSM characteristics of social phobia.

Theoretical models of social phobia mirror those for phobias in general. Preparedness, self-efficacy, and intrapsychic anxiety are viewed as important by different theoretical models.

Cognitive-behavioral therapy has proven successful in treating social phobias. Exposure, relaxation training, and cognitive restructuring have all been shown to be effective for reducing symptoms associated with social phobia. Cognitive restructuring is a technique in which patients are helped to identify, challenge, and modify dysfunctional thoughts. A combination of pharmacological therapy using benzodiazepines such as Librium or Valium, or antidepressant medications with psychological treatments has been proven effective.

Generalized Anxiety Disorder (GAD)

GAD involves anxiety that isn't attached to any specific stimulus or situation. Patients with GAD often report a life-long history of generalized anxiety, with no clearcut onset. It occurs twice as often in women as in men.

While there is some evidence for heritability of GAD, estimates are modest. Most investigators conclude that specific environmental experiences are critical in determining who develops GAD.

Medication is the most common treatment for GAD. Benzodiazepines, such as Librium, Valium, and Xanax are effective in producing short-term reduction in anxiety, lasting one or two weeks. Long-term use is discouraged due to the addictive properties of these drugs. Cognitive-behavioral therapy, combining relaxation training with cognitive restructuring has been shown to be effective. The cognitive restructuring component of this treatment appears to be critical.

Posttraumatic Stress Disorder (PTSD)

PTSD is triggered by a range of life-threatening or personally devastating experiences including war, disasters, and criminal assaults. The symptoms of PTSD may occur immediately after the traumatic event or emerge months, even years, later.

Being exposed to a traumatic event is necessary for the development of PTSD but insufficient by itself. Genetic influences predispose people to developing PTSD. It is thought that this influence sets a threshold and that when a traumatic event pushes the individual over this threshold, PTSD symptoms result.

PTSD patients have distinctly biological differences than other patients. Patients with PTSD show sustained levels of catecholamines, stress hormones that prepare the body for an emergency, and low levels of cortisol, which is important in regulating metabolism. As a result, the ratio of catecholamine to cortisol is twice as high for PTSD patients than it is for patients with other anxiety disorders and from other diagnostic groups. This biological difference may explain the clinical features of constant vigilance and reactivity (due to high catecholamines) and paranoid-type symptoms (due to low cortisol).

More importantly, however, the hyperreactivity of the catecholamine system may be due to irreversible changes in brain mechanisms caused by exposure to severe stress. Severe stress alters three key brain circuits: the locus ceruleus, which regulates brain hormones that prepare for emergencies; the hypothalamus and pituitary gland, which regulate stress-response hormones; and the opioid system, which blunts pain. Thus, a psychosocial event (exposure to trauma) can cause biological changes that, in turn, make us more vulnerable to psychological stressors.

Effective treatment of PTSD symptoms has been reported for antidepressant medications, cognitive-behavioral therapy, and brief psychodynamic psychotherapy. Psychological treatments appear to share a common feature of trying to help the patient recognize and accept thoughts about the traumatic event that had previously been warded off. Cognitive-behavioral treatments do this directly through the use of imaginal exposure, wherein the patient is asked repeatedly to conjure up detailed images of the events associated with the traumatic experience and to focus on these images until the initial anxiety decreases.

Obsessive Compulsive Disorder (OCD)

Individuals with OCD are driven to think about certain topics or perform certain behaviors over and over again in an attempt to relieve anxiety. The most common obsessions involve themes of aggression, dirt and contamination, sex, religion, and doubt. Obsessions differ fundamentally from normal everyday worries in that they cause marked distress and are often associated with fear of loosing control. Two main types of compulsions are cleaning and checking. OCD affects men and women about equally.

There is a greater incidence of psychiatric disorders in relatives of OCD patients particularly greater rates of depression and GAD. This indicates a biological predisposition for OCD to be transmitted within families. Other biological factors seem important. For example, over 50% of people with OCD have tics -- involuntary motor movements, such as eye blinking and making facial grimaces. From 5 to 15% of OCD patients also have Tourette's syndrome, which is characterized by intermittent bodily tics, sounds, and words. Other neurological disorders that frequently co-occur with OCD are Dydenham's chorea, epilepsy, and Parkinson's disease. All of these neurological disorders affect the basal ganglia and particularly the caudate nucleus in the brain. Patients with OCD metabolize glucose more rapidly in the frontal lobe and cingulate pathway (which connects to the basal ganglia) than controls. All together, these data suggest that the basal ganglia and caudate nucleus are disturbed, or "short-circuited," in OCD triggering repetitive actions and abnormal motor movements. These brain areas depend on serotonin, a neurotransmitter. Drugs which increase the amount of serotonin in the brain are the most effective for treating OCD.

The psychodynamic model holds that OCD patients have an anal-erotic personality. People with this personality type are characterized by orderliness, stinginess, and obstinacy. These traits are seen as the result of fixation at the anal stage of personality growth.

The cognitive-behavioral model suggests that the individual with obsessions has a nonspecific, genetic predisposition to experience anxiety. The model further hypothesizes that the individual grows up in an overcontrolling home environment, leading to rigid standards of personal conduct and vulnerability to self-criticism.

Historically, treatment of OCD has been difficult with poor success rates. Significant advances were made in the 1970s with the development of specific cognitive-behavioral methods. The most successful is exposure and response prevention. The patient is exposed to situations that trigger the obsessive thoughts and are prevented from engaging in compulsive actions.

Three drugs have also been shown to have specific effects in treating OCD: Clomipramine, Prozac (fluoxetine) and fluvoxamine. These drugs are antidepressant drugs that reduce symptoms for many patients. However, patients relapse when the drugs are discontinued. Patients treated with a combination of cognitive-behavioral therapy and medication (clomipramine or fluvoxamine) show better maintenance when the drug is withdrawn.

Because of the difficulties in treating OCD, more radical treatments have been tried including psychosurgery. Once such procedure is cingulotomy, which severs the pathway from the frontal lobe to the basal ganglia.

KEY IDEAS AND OBJECTIVES FOR STUDENTS

After reading the chapter, you should be able to answer each of the following:

1. What is the emphasis of the biological in anxiety?

2. What is the emphasis of psychodynamic models of anxiety?

3. How is anxiety viewed from the cognitive-behavioral models?

4. What is the emphasis of the social view of anxiety?

5. What is the difference between fear and anxiety?

6. What are the characteristics and symptoms of Panic Disorder and what are the subtypes?

7. What are the characteristics and symptoms of Agoraphobia?

8. What are the characteristics and symptoms of specific phobias (which used to be called simple phobias)? Which individuals are more vulnerable to becoming phobic?

9. What do people with social phobias dread? How specific is the phobia?

10. What are the characteristics and symptoms of Generalized anxiety disorder (GAD)? What do patients with GAD often report?

11. What are the characteristics and symptoms of Posttraumatic stress disorder (PTSD) and how is it caused?

12. What are obsessions and compulsions? What are the characteristics and symptoms of Obsessive-Compulsive Disorder?

Anxiety Disorders in the Movies

1. High Anxiety (1977, FoxVideo, 94 min). In this Hitchcock parody, Mel Brooks plays the role of psychiatrist with "High Anxiety." The symptoms fit what many would describe as acrophobia, a specific phobia where the person has an irrational fear of heights. One particular scene provides a clear illustration of the physiological, cognitive, and behavioral components of this disorder. When Brooks is to attend the meeting of the American Psychiatric Association, he checks into his hotel to find out that his room has been "mysteriously" moved from the 2nd floor to the 23rd floor. The hotel is an open-air building with glass elevators and hallways that overlook an atrium. The scene shows the types of avoidance and irrational cognitions seen in this disorder as well as the physiological reactions that are typical of a panic attack.

Questions after watching the movie:

1. Given the text's description of the symptoms that are typical for an individual with a diagnosis of simple phobia, how well did the movie do in presenting an accurate portrayal of this disorder? What "errors" (including errors of omission and commission) were made?

2. How did the film deal with the etiology of this disorder? What were the major consistencies (or inconsistencies) with contemporary theories?

3. How did the film deal with the issue of "treatment" or "cure"? What were the major consistencies (or inconsistencies) with contemporary theories?

4. If you were to be a consultant on a "remake" of this film, what advice would you give the director to help make the symptoms, etiology, and treatment more contemporary?

Using Case Studies in Abnormal Behavior by Meyer and Osborne:
The Anxiety Disorders

General Summary

Chapter 3 presents case material on anxiety disorders with specific detailed information for Agoraphobia, Obsessive-Compulsive Disorder, and Posttraumatic Stress Disorder.

The discussion of the cases of Little Hans, Little Albert, and Little Peter, highlights the controversies and debate between psychoanalytic and behavioral writers in the early to mid 1920s. This comparison should help you see how differing perspectives can play important roles in our interpretation of case study information.

Case Comparisons

Agoraphobia: The Case of Agnes. The diagnostic criteria for Agoraphobia are summarized on page 143 of the text. Provide a summary of the specific characteristics of Agnes that support the diagnosis using each of the three criteria. Are any of the criteria questionable? What factors may have led to the development of this problem for Agnes? Which theoretical models are linked to these factors? What treatment options were considered? Which was used?

Obsessive-Compulsive Disorder: The Case of Bess. The diagnostic criteria for OCD are summarized on page 158 of the text. Provide a summary of the specific characteristics of Bess that support the diagnosis using each of the five criteria. Are any of the criteria questionable? What factors may have led to the development of this problem for Bess? Which theoretical models are linked to these factors? What treatment options were considered? Which was used?

Posttraumatic Stress Disorder: The Case of Ryan. The diagnostic criteria for PTSD are summarized on page 152 of the text. Provide a summary of the specific characteristics of Ryan that support the diagnosis using each of the six criteria. Are any of the criteria questionable? What factors may have led to the development of this problem for Ryan? Which theoretical models are linked to these factors? What treatment options were considered? Which was used?

Integrating Perspectives
A Biopsychosocial Model

The Case of Bess: Perspectives on Obsessive-Compulsive Disorder

Biological Factors

•Bess shared many similar traits with her mother. While one cannot determine if these shared traits are due to shared genetics, one cannot rule out the potential role of genetics.

Psychological Factors

•Learning apparently played a large role in Bess' problems. Early on, her mother showed an inordinate concern for cleanliness. This was particularly true for issues related to sexuality.
•Bess' parents divorced when she was 10. Many of her interpersonal problems, particularly relationships with men, may be related to her observations (or lack of observation) of her parent's relationship. Bess' mother showed much distrust of men and may have inadvertently encouraged Bess to be equally distrusting.
•Bess learned early on to avoid unwanted thoughts through ritualistic behavior. For example, she controlled erotic fantasies by focusing her attention on crossword and jigsaw puzzles.

Social Factors

•Religion played a role in Bess' problems. Her faith left her feeling unsure about sexual feelings. Also, she seemed to have difficulty understanding what it meant to be "saved" or to be a "sinner."
•Social factors served to reinforce some of Bess' problematic behavior as she was able to devote more time to her work and studies as a way of avoiding interpersonal contact. Her perfectionism served her well in her work as an accountant.

Sample Multiple-Choice Questions

1. George learned as a child not to express his aggressive sexual and physical impulses, lest he be punished from his parents. As a result, he began to fear these impulses. Freud would say that George developed __________ as a defense against these impulses.
   a. hysterical anxiety
   b. objective anxiety
   c. neurotic anxiety
   d. moral anxiety

2. Russ recently was in a car accident. Shortly thereafter, when Russ was driving, he had a sudden feeling of intense fear. Additionally, his heart was pounding, and he was sweating, trembling, and choking. Russ had a (an) ____________.
   a. agoraphobic reaction
   b. depressive episode
   c. obsessive-compulsive episode
   d. panic attack

3. Stephanie visits a therapist for treatment of her panic attacks. The therapist helps Stephanie realize that she interprets her bodily sensations in a catastrophic way, which increases her anxiety, and increases the likelihood of a panic attack. The therapist follows a ________ of treatment.
   a. biopsychosocial
   b. biological
   c. cognitive-behavioral
   d. person-centered

4. The most effective drug for treating panic disorder is____________.
   a. Xanax
   b. Prozac
   c. Imipramine
   c. no drug therapy is effective

5. Katie was diagnosed with a panic disorder with agoraphobia. Her husband spends more time with her, taking over many of her responsibilities. He feels he can't be angry with her or he will seem uncaring. By acting this way, he ultimately encourages her dependency and agoraphobia. The ______ model would postulate that this is one example of how panic disorder is developed and maintained.
   a. family systems
   b. cognitive-behavioral
   c. person-centered
   d. psychodynamic

6. A fear of one or more social or performance situations in which the person is exposed to unfamiliar people or possible scrutiny by others is termed _____________.
   a. a specific phobia
   b. social phobia
   c. a complex phobia
   d. agoraphobia

7. Lori seeks treatment for her PTSD after being raped at gun point last year. Her therapist asks Lori to repeatedly conjure up detailed images surrounding the rape and focus on these details until the anxiety decreases. This treatment is called _________.
   a. systematic desensitization
   b. imaginal exposure
   c. cognitive restructuring
   d. relaxation training

8. Levi is anxious. Every few weeks his anxiety reaches a point where Levi feels he has to do something. When this happens, he shops because it is the only thing that relieves his anxiety. On his shopping binges, he buys things he doesn't want or need. The repetitive, anxious thoughts and impulses that Levi has are _____________.
   a. obsessions
   b. compulsions
   c. delusions
   d. abreactions

9. A cognitive-behavioral perspective on treatment of OCD has two parts. The first part, ____________, is when touching or handling items that trigger certain compulsions is required. The second part, __________, is when the compulsive behavior is not allowed to happen.
   a. response-prevention, exposure
   b. exposure, response-prevention
   c. flooding, desensitization
   d. flooding, exposure

10. Robert has had persistent, pervasive anxiety for about 13 months in a number of different situations. He has also suffered from shakiness, racing heart, inability to relax, an exaggerated startle response, insomnia, light-headedness, and irritability. He is best diagnosed as having ______disorder.
    a. panic
    b. phobic
    c. obsessive-compulsive
    d. generalized anxiety

Answer Key

1. c
2. d
3. c
4. c
5. a
6. b
7. b
8. a
9. b
10. d

CHAPTER 6 - SOMATOFORM AND DISSOCIATIVE DISORDERS

This chapter begins with a detailed summary of the Case of Anna O. Anna O. was a 21-year-old woman treated by Josef Breuer using a technique that he labeled as a "talking cure." This type of therapy provided the foundation for psychoanalysis, and the Case of Anna O. was discussed extensively by Sigmund Freud as a foundation for his psychoanalytic theory of neurosis. This chapter examines Anna O's symptoms as they related to the diagnostic criteria for somatoform and dissociative disorders.

Somatoform Disorders

Somatoform disorders are characterized by symptoms typically associated with physical diseases, without a known organic basis for the symptoms. Thus, these symptoms are linked to psychological processes. The 5 DSM-IV somatoform disorders are: conversion disorder, somatization disorder, hypochondriasis, body dysmorphic disorder, and pain disorder.

Conversion Disorders

Anna O. is the classic example used to illustrate conversion disorders. Historically, these disorders were called hysterical neuroses. The term hysteria comes from the Greek word meaning uterus. This reflects the early view that these disorders could be linked to problems when a woman does not have sexual relationships or is childless. It was hypothesized that the uterus would "wander" throughout the body and the symptoms would be linked to "where" the uterus was lodged. Contemporary research is inconsistent with this perspective. Men account for some 20 - 40% of all diagnosed cases of conversion disorders.

Symptoms associated with conversion disorders develop quickly, usually under severe psychological stress. Individuals with a history of hysterical or dependent personality disorder may be at greater risk for the development of these disorders though there is no clear link between these disorders. Incidence rates were higher in the late nineteeth century than today.

It is critical to distinguish conversion disorder from malingering and factitious disorders, but difficult to determine. Malingering differs from conversion disorder in that the individual is intentionally faking symptoms in order to obtain some reward or to avoid some unpleasant situation. Factitious disorder involves the purposeful production of symptoms. For example, individuals with Munchausen syndrome appears motivated to play a "sick role" and actively seeks out hospitalization to treat symptoms that they have induced.

The validity of conversion disorder has been debated. One classic study found that 21 of 85 patients diagnosed with conversion disorder eventually developed acute physical illnesses consistent with their symptoms. Thus, in some cases, conversion disorder may be the result of an inaccurate physical diagnosis.

The Psychodynamic model is the only well developed theory of conversion disorder. The key assumption of this model is that the symptoms keep intrapsychic anxiety or conflict from awareness. This unconscious anxiety is converted into a physical problem and the symptoms are symbolic of the intrapsychic conflict. The case of Anna O was presented by Freud as illustrative of the effectiveness of the "talking cure" (the basic foundation of psychoanalysis) for treating conversion disorders. Conceptually, the cure come about through a process known as catharsis wherein the individual experiences relief from disclosing emotionally charged thoughts and feelings.

The text points out, however, that the case of Anna O did not end as successfully as Freud indicated. Rather, she suffered many relapses and was institutionalized for almost two years. She became addicted to a drug that Breuer had prescribed (chloral hydrate) and to morphine given during her hospitalization. Breuer was aware of this failure and reported that he had hopes that she might die and be released from her suffering.

Freud and Breuer developed quite different perspectives about the role of sexual conflict as a cause of conversion disorder. Over time, Freud began to believe that all conversion disorders were the result of unresolved sexual conflict. Breuer felt that while sexual conflicts were important, they were not the root of every case. Modern psychodynamic theory is more in accord with Breuer than Freud.

One problem with the psychodynamic explanation of conversion disorder is that this theory predicts that patients with conversion disorder should show no anxiety. This lack of anxiety, referred to as la belle indifference, has not been supported by research. Rather, individuals with conversion disorder typically show more anxiety than normal controls. In addition, conversion symptoms are often associated with overt expression of anxiety.

The behavioral model suggests that conversion disorder is related to the adoption of social roles whereby behavior matches symptoms of a physical disease. Behavioral research has shown that people are responsive to demand characteristics in social situations and that individuals with conversion disorder must have had experience with the symptom which results in some type of reinforcement of the behaviors associated with the symptoms.

The behavioral model does not differentiate between conversion disorder and malingering. This distinction is seen as a nonissue. The rationale is that they do not differentiate between conscious and unconscious processes. The major shortcoming of this model is that it is more a description of the disorder than an explanation. The model does not explain how or why individuals develop this disorder in response to psychological stress.

Somatization Disorder

Somatization disorder is characterized by a pattern of recurrent, long-standing somatic symptoms, beginning before age 30 and occurring over a period of several years. Research suggests that the number of symptoms present may be important in determining severity of the disorder. Specifically, individuals with 9 to 12 symptoms seem equally disturbed as individuals with 13 or more symptoms. For both of these groups, the presence of anxiety and major depressive disorders were comparable, but far more common in these groups than in patients with fewer than 6 somatic symptoms.

Other psychological disorders are often identified in patients diagnosed with somatization disorder, particularly anxiety and depression. Suicide attempts, interpersonal difficulties, and antisocial behaviors are common.

The major explanatory model for this disorder is the biopsychosocial model. Research suggests a biological predisposition for developing this disorder. Women with this disorder are more likely to have a family member who has been similarly diagnosed or first-degree relatives diagnosed as antisocial personality disorder. Some have suggested that gender issues influence the expression of this disorder with women more likely to have symptoms consistent with somatization disorder and men more likely to have symptoms consistent with antisocial personality disorder.

Cultural factors seem to play an important role in the expression of symptoms associated with somatitization disorders. The text points out the fact that while the prevalence of this disorder is decreasing, the incidence of women engaged in antisocial acts or problems associated with borderline personality disorder are increasing. The general conclusion is that cultural factors influence the behavioral expression of particular underlying predispositions.

Patients with somatitization disorder have health care costs 9 times the national average. Much of this is due to unnecessary hospitalizations. While the cost is high, there is no evidence that the costs associated with treatment help. Research has shown that when physicians are provided detailed information about this disorder, costs can be better controlled. Specifically, physicians are instructed to schedule appointments every 4 to 6 weeks, to be careful to not convey the idea that the patients' complaints are merely psychological, and to minimize the use of unnecessary hospitalizations, laboratory tests, and surgery unless clearly indicated. This treatment did not help reduce the somatitization symptoms, however, medical costs decreased substantially.

Hypochondriasis

In hypochondriasis, an individual fears that he or she has a serious physical illness, dispute medical evidence to the contrary. Research suggests that individuals with this disorder often experience a range of other psychological problems, the most common being anxiety and mood disorders. The psychodynamic model suggests that individuals with hypochondriasis focus on somatic concerns so that "real" anxieties remain unconscious.

A detailed illustration of misinterpretations of bodily sensations is provided to illustrate how a cognitive model would account for the development of hypochondriasis. This model was also presented in Chapter 5 and is illustrative of how both panic disorders and hypochondriasis develop. First, these individuals misinterpret bodily sensations (such as a lump in the throat) as indicating ill health. Second, they perceive the symptoms as leading to irreparable physical harm. Third, individuals with hypochondriasis develop a pattern of checking their bodies and constantly seeking consultation from physicians.

Body Dysmorphic Disorder

Individuals with this disorder are preoccupied with an imaginary defect in physical appearance. These individuals are often preoccupied with excessive facial hair or the shape of their nose, mouth, or jaw. In all cases, the concern is greatly exaggerated. This disorder typically begins in adolescence or early childhood and is common among both men and women.

Pain Disorder

Individuals with pain disorders may have pain associated with psychological factors or psychological factors combined with a general medical condition. The essential feature is the presence of pain that cannot be better accounted for by purely physical reasons. This disorder occurs more frequently in women than in men.

Dissociative Disorders

These disorders are characterized by change in the normal, integrated functions of the person's identity, memory, or consciousness. Four dissociative disorders are identified in the DSM-IV: Dissociative amnesia, dissociative fugue, depersonalization disorder, and dissociative identity disorder.

Dissociative Amnesia

This disorder is characterized by a sudden loss of memory for important personal information, not due to an organic problem. The most common forms are localized amnesia (specific period of time) and selective amnesia (loss of memory for some, but not all events in a specific period of time). Less common are generalized amnesia (memory loss of one's entire life) and continuous amnesia (total memory loss following a specific point in time).

Severe psychological stress appears to be the cause of dissociative amnesia. The symptoms appears suddenly, and often disappear quickly with complete recovery and rare recurrence.

Dissociative Fugue

Individuals with a dissociative fugue experience symptoms such as traveling away from home, taking on a new identity, and failing to remember these actions after recovery. This disorder is quite rare.

Depersonalization Disorder

Depersonalization disorder is characterized by an individual having the sense of being an outside observer of his or her own thoughts and feelings. While experiencing depersonalization, the person often feels that he or she is not in full control and this feeling often causes severe personal distress. This disorder usually begins in adolescence and indications are that some 70 percent of young adults may experience brief periods of depersonalization. The number of individuals with symptoms severe enough to warrant diagnosis is unknown.

Dissociative Identity Disorder

Dissociative identity disorder is the new term for multiple-personality disorder. Individuals with dissociative identity disorder experience two or more distinct personalities that take turns controlling the actions of the individual. In the process of these distinct personalities taking control, the individual experiences an inability to recall important personal information.

The most famous case of dissociative identity disorder is the case of Chris Costner Sizemore, the subject of the famous book The Three Faces of Eve by Thigpen and Cleckley. In this case, three personalities were described. Eve White was a sweet, conservative, inhibited woman who was a hard-worker and devoted mother who sought treatment for blackouts. Eve Black was the opposite of Eve White. This second personality was seductive and impulsive. Eve White was allergic to nylon stockings, Eve Black had no allergy. During treatment, a third personality developed. This personality, known as Jane was more self-confident and spontaneous than Eve White.

While the number of distinct personalities necessary for the diagnosis of dissociative identity disorder is 2, the DSM-IV points out that almost half of the recently reported cases have 10 or more personalities. A major problem in determining the number of personalities is that the number changes over time and through the course of treatment. Autobiographical reports from Ms. Sizemore indicate that she developed several more distinct personalities after treatment ended.

While the onset of this disorder is almost always during childhood, the disorder does not typically come to the attention of mental health professionals until the individual is an adolescent or adult. Research suggests that these individuals have many additional serious problems. It is common that individuals with dissociative identity disorder have a history of mental health treatment, hospitalizations, suicide attempts, and sexual abuse.

The chapter presents detailed explanations of the cause of dissociative identity disorder from four perspectives: Psychodynamic, behavioral, cognitive, and biological. The psychodynamic model suggests that dissociation is a means to keep painful events out of consciousness. The feelings of pain become entrenched as separate personalities. There is considerable evidence that individuals with dissociative identity disorder have a history of serious childhood abuse. In addition, individuals prone to dissociative identity disorder are very suggestible and easy to hypnotize. This capacity presumably helps individuals separate themselves from early traumatic experiences. Individuals who cannot dissociate easily may resort to defense mechanisms such as denial or repression to protect themselves.

The behavioral model suggests that individuals with dissociative identity disorder are actually playing social roles that were learned through modeling or exposure to information about given disorders. These roles are maintained by reinforcement of their behavior. In addition, the behavioral model suggests that given proper encouragement, many suggestible individuals can take on alternate personalities. The text points out that this model is good at describing dissociative identity disorder, but fails to explain this disorder.

The cognitive model focuses on the significance of state dependent memory. That is, individuals remember events best when they are experiencing a mood state similar to the mood state when learning occurred. Specifically, during happy moods, people remember happy events, while during sad moods, people remember sad events better. In addition to state dependent memory, the mood congruity effect suggests that individuals selectively focus on material that is consistent with their current mood state.

The biological model is not well developed. There are suggestions that dissociative symptoms are more common for individuals with other disorders (such as PTSD), and there is a suggestion that there are similar biological factors responsible for both disorders. Finally, it has been suggested that dissociation might be linked to brain mechanisms, however, this theory is not well developed.

The most common treatments for dissociative identity disorders are hypnosis and psychodynamic psychotherapy. Siegel has suggested specific goals of treatment that involve direct confrontation of traumatic experiences and support. However there are few controlled treatment outcome studies.

KEY IDEAS AND OBJECTIVES FOR STUDENTS

After reading the chapter, you should be able to answer the following questions:

1. What are the characteristics of individuals with somatoform disorders?

2. What symptoms do individuals with conversion disorder develop? If no physical illness is misdiagnosed, what explains these symptoms?

3. What are the characteristics and symptoms of somatization disorder?

4. What are the characteristics and symptoms of hypochondriasis? With what other problems in this disorder strongly associated?

5. What are the characteristics and symptoms of body dysmorphic disorder?

6. What are the characteristics and symptoms of individuals with pain disorder?

7. What are the characteristics of the dissociative disorders?

8. What are the characteristics and symptoms of dissociative amnesia?

9. What are the characteristics and symptoms of dissociative fugue? What typically triggers them and how long do they last?

10. What are the characteristics and symptoms of individuals with dissociative identity disorder (formerly known as multiple personality disorder)?

Somatoform and Dissociative Disorders in the Movies

Films illustrating Dissociative Identity Disorder:

1. Three Faces of Eve (Fox Video, 1957, 91 min). This film is based on Thigpen & Cleckley's 1954 book and portrays the case of Chris Costner Sizemore. Three distinct personalities are presented, as well as the use of hypnosis in her treatment.

2. Sybil (Fox Video, 1976, 122 min). This made-for-TV movie is based on the book of the same name which explores the life of a woman with 17 distinct personalities. The role of childhood trauma and reintegration therapy are presented.

3. Primal Fear (not on video at this time). This recent film focuses on the issue of personal responsibility in a case of dissociative identity disorder. Ironically, after winning the case, the defense lawyer learns that his client had only pretended to have the disorder. The movie highlights the controversy between psychiatric disorders and legal issues and can also be used for discussion of the insanity defense in Chapter 21.

Students should identify the characteristics of dissociative identity disorder as presented in the text, and compare them with those presented in the movies. What aspects of therapy were demonstrated in the film(s)? How might the use of hypnosis (as presented in the movie) have influenced the number of personalities demonstrated (i.e., could these personalities have emerged as the result of hypnosis or were they merely revealed and reintegrated through hypnosis?).

Films illustrating Somatoform Disorders

1. Joe vs. the Volcano (Warner, 1990, 106 min). This film opens with the main character "Joe" displaying behaviors consistent with hypochondriasis. He spends a great deal of time talking to co-workers about his symptoms and is sure that he will die. The opening scene is an excellent example of the debilitating effects of this disorder.

2. Annie Hall (MGM/United Artists, 1977, 94 min) This film illustrates symptoms associated with somatization in several spots, but the most clear example comes when Woody Allen's character is to receive an award. The stress associated with this event overwhelms him and he develops a range of somatic symptoms with no observable cause. In one scene, he is lying in bed with a physician examining him while Diane Keaton is on the phone with the organizers of the award. The physician tries to get Woody Allen to eat something, but he can't. Diane Keaton gets off the phone and informs Woody Allen that the award presentation has been canceled. She then begins a conversation with the physician while Woody Allen starts to feel so much better that he begins to eat in the background.

Students are encouraged to watch these two movies and consider the differences and similarities of different somatoform disorders. Also, the movies provide a good example to the differences between public perception of psychologically based physical symptoms and actually symptoms of the disorders.

Using <u>Case Studies in Abnormal Behavior</u> by Meyer and Osborne:
The Somatoform Disorders

This chapter briefly reviews the somatoform disorders by outlining the 4 disorders in this category (Somatization Disorder, Conversion Disorder, Psychogenic Pain Disorder, and Hypochondriasis). The major symptoms are described and issues related to the development of the disorder and accurate diagnosis are presented. The chapter focuses on Psychogenic Pain Disorder and provides an in-depth case study of Pam. Different treatment options are explored to illustrate the different theoretical approaches to this disorder. Finally, the treatment approach used with Pam is reviewed, which used a multidisciplinary approach and which included her husband in treatment.

Suggestions:

1. Compare the 4 disorders in this category and make a list of the similarities and differences among the 4 types.

2. Evaluate Pam's history from the perspective of the psychodynamic, behavioral, and biopsychosocial models. Which theory best captures and explains the development and course of Pam's disorder?

3. Examine the multidisciplinary treatment of Pam from each of the theoretical perspectives presented in the text. How well does the treatment (or different components of the treatment) fit with each of these perspectives? Does the success of the treatment have implications for which perspective is supported?

Integrating Perspectives
A Biopsychosocial Model

Use the Case of Pam to demonstrate the biopsychosocial model and the interactive effects of biological, psychological, and social factors.

Biological Factors

•Pam had experienced pain since her early teens that she linked to a real auto accident that occurred when she was 18. However, the role of physiological factors were never supported by medial examinations.
•Her migraine headaches also were not consistent with the typical migraine pattern.

Psychological Factors

•Pam was the second youngest of 4 children. Her father worked hard and was rarely at home. Pam viewed her parents as cool and aloof, rarely showing affection.
•Pam's mother was very protective of the father and was critical when the children expressed any complaints about the father not being around much. However, she suspected that her mother also resented the father's absence, but could not express this directly.
•Pam's mother, like Pam, experienced "medical" problems that required that she say off her feet for a few days. During this time, Pam's father would give her mother a great deal of attention until she was well again and then he would throw himself back into his work to "catch up."

Social Factors

•Pam views male and female roles in a traditional fashion with the woman's role in the home and the man's role as the breadwinner. The family has moved several times to enhance her husband's work. However, she is resistant to another move and discussion of moving seem to bring on headaches.

Sample Multiple-Choice Questions

1. During a psychotherapy session, John expresses a great deal of anger that he has had towards his father for many years. Afterwards, he feels a sense of relief. This psychological relief that accompanies expression of emotionally charged thoughts and feelings is called __________.
   a. hysteria
   b. catharsis
   c. transference
   d. dissociation

2. In 1964, Jane Smith was diagnosed as having a hysterical neurosis. If she were to present with these same symptoms today, it is likely that she would be diagnosed with __________.
   a. hypochondriasis
   b. conversion disorder
   c. histrionic personality disorder
   d. dissociative identity disorder

3. Somatization disorder was formerly known as ________.
   a. la belle indifference
   b. malingering
   c. Briquet's syndrome
   d. cathartic disorder

4. Andrea frequently finds herself thinking about illnesses. When she begins to think about an illness that she might have she begins to ruminate or worry constantly about bodily sensations and wonders if they are related to this possible illness. Her worries continue until she sees her physician. After the visit, she feels better for a few days, but often begins to worry about a new sensation and what illness might be related to this sensation. Andrea's behaviors are similar to those of individuals diagnosed as having ____________.
   a. somatization disorder
   b. conversion disorder
   c. hypochondriasis
   d. Munchausen's syndrome

5. ________ disorder involves the sense of being an outside observer of one's own thoughts and feelings.
   a. Depersonalization
   b. Dissociative identity
   c. Dissociative fugue
   d. Dissociative amnesia

6. When the normal, integrated function of a person's identity or consciousness undergoes a sudden change, he or she is most likely suffering from __________.
   a. a dissociative disorder
   b. malingering
   c. a somatoform disorder
   d. an anxiety disorder

7. The case of Mr. M., the man who was found lying in the road without any memory of himself or his past, and who had been raped, was suffering from __________ disorder.
   a. dissociative fugue
   b. dissociative amnesia
   c. depersonalization
   d. dissociative identity disorder

8. Which of the following statements is true of people experiencing dissociative fugue?
   a. they frequently display violent behavior
   b. after recovering their original identity, they are able to remember the full events occurring during their dissociative fugue state
   c. the disorder is quite common and is usually precipitated by minor stressors
   d. the age of onset is variable

9. Depersonalization disorder is different from the other dissociative disorders because in depersonalization __________.
   a. there are no perceptual disturbances
   b. there are no memory disturbances
   c. there is no anxiety or distress experienced
   d. the person loses contact with reality

10. Which of the following factors contributes to the difficulty in accurately diagnosing dissociative identity disorder?
    a. the different personalities or identities are usually in conflict with one another
    b. few individuals report memory lapses
    c. some of the symptoms may appear to be symptoms of schizophrenia
    d. individuals with dissociative identity disorder are difficult to hypnotize, so it is difficult to gain access to all the separate identities

Answer Key

1. b
2. b
3. c
4. c
5. a
6. a
7. b
8. d
9. b
10. c

CHAPTER 7 MOOD DISORDERS

Description

Mood disorders are characterized primarily by disturbances in mood and are quite common. Major depression (the "common cold of mental illness"), bipolar disorders, and other forms of depression and mania, occur in episodes (discrete periods of time in which a number of specified symptoms are present, representing a change from previous functioning).

Major Depressive Episodes. Depressive symptoms can be primary or can occur in connection with other disorders. Three primary features are: 1) persistent mood disturbance by depressed mood and anhedonia (marked loss of interest or pleasure in activities); 2) somatic symptoms including appetite or weight changes, sleep problems, psychomotor agitation (marked increase in physical restlessness), and psychomotor retardation (significant slowing down of motor activity); and 3) cognitive symptoms including feelings of worthlessness, excessive inappropriate guilt, greatly increased difficulty in thinking or concentrating, and recurrent thoughts of death or suicide. Specifiers describe subtypes of mood disorders. They are designed to assist in treatment selection and to improve predictions of the course and outcome of the disorder. Melancholic features refer to a particularly severe episode characterized by almost complete loss of pleasure and reactivity to positive stimuli, early morning awakening with worse feelings of depression in the morning, and less ability to identify stressors which triggered the episode. Biological treatments are more likely to be effective for melancholic depression. Atypical features refer to a subtype characterized by mood reactivity to positive stimuli, weight gain or increased appetite, hypersomnia, leaden paralysis, and extreme sensitivity to interpersonal rejection; particular types of antidepressant medication are more likely to be effective. Seasonal pattern refers to a subtype known as seasonal affective disorder, in which symptoms appear in winter and disappear in the spring, even without treatment; exposure to light is an effective treatment for this subtype, which occurs more among young people and those in northern latitudes.

Manic episodes are characterized by extremely elevated mood and related changes in behavior and physical and cognitive functioning. These are evident by animated and impulsive behavior, and persons may exhibit constant motion, loud and incessant talking, grandiose ideas, buying sprees, or unrestrained sexual activity. The mania represents the primary symptoms of mood disturbance, although the mood is bipolar or opposite to depression. The manic mood is often very labile or changeable. Somatic symptoms include psychomotor agitation (with a hyperactive, excessive quality), and decreased need for sleep. Cognitive symptoms include pressured speech (loud, fast, nonstop talking that is hard to direct or interrupt), and flight of ideas (thoughts or speech that jumps from topic to topic with no clear direction or plan). Distractibility and poor judgment often accompany manic episodes, which tend to develop more quickly and to be briefer in duration than depressive episodes.

Hypomanic episodes are shorter, milder versions of manic episodes which do not require hospitalization or cause marked impairment in functioning. The symptoms are identical to those of mania, except that they are not as severe or long-lasting. A mixed episode is characterized by alternation between full-blown depressive and manic episodes. Prognosis is poorest for this type.

Types of Mood Disorders

Table 7.1 on page 197 lists the major types of mood disorders in DSM-IV. Major Depressive disorder, single episode, refers to a single major depressive episode without a history of manic, hypomanic, or mixed episodes. Major Depressive disorder, recurrent is diagnosed when the episode is not the first instance. Unipolar refers to major depression. Bipolar refers to Manic, Mixed, or Hypomanic depression. Bipolar I disorder is diagnosed when the patient is experiencing or has had one or more manic or mixed episodes, usually alternating with major depressive episodes. The specifier, rapid cycling is used if four or more episodes occur within one year. Bipolar II disorder is diagnosed when the patient is experiencing or has a history of one or more major depressive and hypomanic episodes, but has never had a manic or mixed episode. The specifier, with atypical features, is used when mixed or major depressive episode shows the particular symptoms associated with this subtype.

Dysthymic Disorder is characterized by relatively chronic depressed mood that is less severe but is longer lasting than major depression. Loss of energy, feelings of hopeless and low self-esteem are specific criteria. Psychomotor disturbance and suicidal ideation do NOT occur with this type. Double depression occurs when a major depressive episodes occurs in combination with dysthymia, and is associated with a poorer prognosis than a single depressive disorder. Cyclothymic disorder is characterized by a period of 2 or more years in which hypomanic symptoms alternate with depressive symptoms that are less severe than those in a major depressive episode (so bipolar II criteria are not met).

Issues and Problems

Major depression is the single most common psychiatric disorder in the U.S. Point prevalence is the percentage of the population who have the disorder at a particular time or over a given period. The point prevalence rate over a 12-month period in the U.S. is: 8% for men and 13% for women for major depression; 2.1% for men and 3% for women for dysthymia; 1.4% for men and 1.3% for women for manic episode. Lifetime prevalence is the percentage of individuals who have ever had a specific disorder at any time. Lifetime prevalence rates for the U.S. are: 12.7% for men and 21.3% for women for major depressive episode; 4.8% for men and 8% for women for dysthymia; and 1.6% for men and 1.7% for women for manic episode. A risk factor is a variable that increases a person's tendency to develop a disorder. Gender is a risk factor for depression, but not for manic episodes. The *Thinking About Gender Issues* box on page 203 explores theories to account for this risk factor. Other possible risk factors include age, income, and race/ethnicity. However, depression is NOT found more among the elderly; prevalence is highest in 18- to 24-year-old men and 25- to 44-year-old women, and adolescents. Income also is NOT related to depression; depression is more likely to occur in those at the extreme low end of the income scale, but otherwise does not vary with income level. It also is not clear how and/or to what extent race/ethnicity affects mood disorders; with a few exceptions, whites have higher rates.

Comorbidity is the co-occurrence of two or more disorders. It occurs most often in mood disorders because the disorders share features ranging from underlying genetic factors to demographic risk factors to environmental stressors. There is approximately 50% overlap between anxiety and depression. Recovery is more difficult in these cases and the risk of suicide may be higher (e.g., panic disorder).

Other mood disorders fall under the category Mood Disorder NOS. These include premenstrual dysphoric disorder, more commonly known as PMS. Minor depressive disorder is diagnosed when fewer than 5 criteria for major depressive disorder are met. Brief recurrent depressive disorder is diagnosed when the criteria for major depressive disorder have been present for less than 2 weeks.

Depression is the most common factor leading to suicide; approximately 90% of those committing suicide have a psychological disorder and 45-70% of them have a mood disorder. About 15% of those with mood disorders eventually commit suicide. Approximately 30,000 persons commit suicide each year in the U.S., and about 300,000 attempt suicide. Women make twice as many suicide attempts, but men succeed in killing themselves 3-4 times as often due to their use of more lethal methods. Suicide attempts are most common among young people, but completed suicides increase with age. Twenty-five percent of all suicides occur in those over 65. The second-leading cause of death among 15- to 24-year-olds, however, is suicide, pointing to the increase among the young. Whites have twice as many suicides overall, but certain nonwhite groups are at especial risk for suicide (e.g., inner-city African Americans, female physicians). Those with bipolar mood disorders have higher risk than unipolar disorder persons. Reasons for committing suicide vary, but are often linked to hopelessness which leads the individual to perceive suicide as their only solution. *Table 7.2* on page 207 presents common reasons for suicide. Approximately 80% of those who commit suicide give warnings of their intentions, such as verbalizing their intentions, preparing a will, etc. Risk factors for suicide include anxiety and depression, and a family history of suicide.

Causes

Biological factors. Genetic factors have been supported by family, twin, and adoption studies. Research suggests that unipolar depression is passed on within families, and perhaps an additional problem is unique to bipolar disorder. The more severe the depression in a subject, the more likely it is that relatives will develop a mood disorder. The concordance rate for major depression is 40% in monozygotic twins and only 10% for dizygotic twins. The concordance rate for bipolar disorder is 70-80% for monozygotic twins, but only 10-20% for dizygotic twins. Adoption studies, which provide control for similarity of environment, also support the role of genetic factors. More mood disorders occur in the biological relatives of those with mood disorders; this is true for both unipolar and bipolar disorders. The severity of the mood disorder appears to be related to the strength of the genetic loading. The means by which vulnerability to mood disorders is transmitted has yet to be determined.

Neurobiochemical factors which may be linked to mood disorders include neurotransmitters and neuroendocrine abnormalities. Neurotransmitters may be affected by antidepressant medications; medication may interfere with the reuptake process (reabsorption of the neurotransmitter into the neuron from which it was released) and/or interfere with the process in which neurotransmitters are broken down chemically in the synapse into simpler compounds by monoamine oxidase. Imbalances in norepinephrine, serotonin, and dopamine, may occur when homeostatic mechanisms that work to keep the system in a steady state, including steady sensitivity of postsynaptic receptors malfunction. This may be related to mood disorders. Presynaptic receptors involve multiple neurotransmitters and neuropeptides. This process is very complex, making it difficult to determine how mood disorders develop. Certain endocrine diseases, such as hypothyroidism and Cushing's syndrome have been linked to depression. High cortisol levels have been monitored with the dexamethasone suppression test (DST), which has Been used to predict response to treatment. Sleep dysfunction in the form of less deep (slow-wave) sleep, earlier onset of rapid eye movement sleep and increased amounts of REM sleep have been found in depressed individuals. Serotonin and norepinephrine are involved in REM sleep and may be linked to the sleep abnormalities in depressed individuals.

Psychosocial factors include psychodynamic, cognitive, and interpersonal factors. Psychodynamic models have emphasized the role of interpersonal relationships and loss of love and emotional security. Freud hypothesized that anger at a lost lover was turned inward, which led to depression. Revised hypotheses have examined dependency as it relates to anger. Self-esteem loss has received more attention, especially in conjunction with stressful life events, unstable sense of self, and few external sources of self-worth. Self-criticism and achievement-related stressors have also been studied. Empirical studies have provided only partial support for these factors.

Beck's cognitive distortion model has been very influential in the study of depression. He hypothesized that individuals with depression exhibit distortions of reality and depressogenic cognitions which cause depression. Negative automatic thoughts are accepted by the depressed individual, which include arbitrary inferences, overgeneralization, and magnification and minimization. Beck hypothesized that beliefs and knowledge about ourselves are organized into a schema that filters and organizes experiences. Depressed people have a cognitive triad of negative schema, which involves a negative view of the self, the world, and the future. Depressed person's automatic thoughts also show content specificity by focusing on experiences of loss and failure. Research has supported the presence of distorted, automatic cognitions in depressed people, but the causal relationship of these factors to depression has yet to be established.

Seligman's learned helplessness model is an attributional model of depression. He proposed that those who were exposed to uncontrollable aversive situations would develop depression that was rooted in feelings of helplessness that affects their interpretation of causes of events in their lives. This attributional style (cognitive style regarding beliefs about the causes of events) is characterized by internal (attribute negative events to own failings), stable (belief that causes of negative events remains constant), and global (assume causes of negative events have broad and general effects) attributions. Research which failed to support the theory that a hopeless attributional styles causes depression led to a revised model, the hopelessness theory of depression. This is a diathesis-stress model in which a person with a cognitive vulnerability (diathesis) experiences a negative life event (the stress), then makes negative, stable, and global attributions about its cause; this would then lead to hopelessness depression. While research supports this model as an accurate description of some aspects of depression, it cannot account for the cause of depression.

Self-focus can lead to negative emotions because it initiates a self-evaluative process which can end in self-criticism. Those with mild depression have high levels of self-focus and self-focus increases following loss. Women self-focus more than do men; if this becomes persistent, a ruminative response style could enhance memory bias for negative experiences, interfere with concentration, and interfere with complex thinking and problem solving. These could serve to maintain depression. Others have theorized that depressed individuals lack positive thinking. The tripartite model stems from this and compares depression and anxiety. Negative affectivity is a temperamental sensitivity to negative stimuli and predisposes one to develop an anxiety disorder, a mood disorder, or both. In anxiety, individuals exhibit a specific personality factor which consists of the physical symptoms that accompany an anxious mood. In depression, individuals exhibit a deficit in a specific personality factor called positive affectivity; they are less sensitive to rewards and are less likely to experience positive emotions. Both depressed and anxious patients have high negativity, which accounts for their co-occurrence. Depressed individuals have specifically depressive thoughts (focused on loss) and low positive affectivity. These and other temperament dimensions are being linked to underlying biological systems, such as the behavioral inhibition system, the behavioral activation system, and the fight-or-flight system.

Interpersonal factors have been studied by neo-Freudians Harry Stack Sullivan and Erik Erikson. Lack of social support has been associated with depression, and longitudinal studies suggest that this is a causal factor in depression. Marital discord also co-occurs with depression. The *Thinking About Social Issues* box on page 218 explores the gender differences in depression and marital satisfaction. Coyne's interactional perspective on depression hypothesizes that the needs and demands of people who are depressed place a strain on their interpersonal relationships; their depressive behaviors of social skills deficits, negativity, and interpersonal distance may lead to a vicious cycle which exacerbates and/or maintains depression.

The biopsychosocial approach also uses a diathesis-stress model in which a biological vulnerability (diathesis) interacts with life stressors. This interaction may occur through lowered immune functioning, and neurotransmitter dysfunction. The *Integrating Perspectives: A Biopsychosocial Model* box on page 220 illustrates this model more fully. Although manic phases were once thought to be solely biological in nature, more recent research has suggested that psychological factors, such as life stressors, may also be important.

Treatment

Biological therapies include medications, electroconvulsive treatment (ECT), and light therapy. Tricyclic antidepressants are the oldest drugs used with depression. Fifty to sixty percent of patients with major depression show improvement in symptoms, while only 25-30% show improvement with placebos. Side effects include dry mouth, constipation, blurred vision, and difficulty urinating. Tricyclic antidepressants initially increase available neurotransmitters by blocking synaptic reuptake and it takes several weeks for adjustment of the postsynaptic receptors and for improvement in symptoms. Selective serotonin reuptake inhibitors (SSRIs) are drugs specific to serotonin and do not affect other transmitters. Prozac was the first widely known drug of this class. Research suggests that SSRIs are as effective as tricyclics in reducing depression, produce fewer side effects, are NOT associated with increased violence, suicide, or suicide attempts, have lower risk of fatal overdose, and may be effective for treating dysthymic disorder that has not responded to psychotherapy. Monoamine oxidase inhibitors (MAOIs) slow the rate of chemical breakdown of neurotransmitters at the synapse and work best for patients with atypical depressive features (mood reactivity, increased sleep and appetite, leaden paralysis, and rejection sensitivity), and those with features of personality disorder. While they are about as effective in reducing depressive symptoms as other antidepressant medications, severe hypertension and death can result if they are taken with food or drink containing the amino acid tyramine (found in cheese, alcohol, chocolate). Lithium is effective with bipolar I, bipolar II, and severe cyclothymia. Approximately 50-80% of bipolar I patients report full or partial reduction of both manic and depressive episodes; however, treatment may need to be long-term (2 years) to prevent relapse. Lithium is also effective with recurrent unipolar disorder. Side effects include gastric distress, weight gain, tremor and fatigue. Toxic levels of lithium are also close to therapeutic levels.

Electroconvulsive therapy (ECT) is very controversial and involves using electrical charges to the brain to induce a generalized seizure. It is most often used for those who are seriously depressed (e.g., highly suicidal) who require quicker treatment than drugs, those with psychotic features to depression that do not respond well to medication alone, and those in acute manic episodes. About 80% of depressed patients show improvement with ECT, and ECT may act more quickly than lithium in bipolar patients. Initial ECT was problematic: patients were awake during seizures, which were frightening and painful, bone fractures resulted from motor activity during seizures, and bilateral placement of electrodes led to serious memory impairment. Current practice involves general anesthetics and muscle relaxants, and unilateral placement of electrodes to reduce memory impairment. Most show improvement after a few treatments. Memory impairment is common, but usually remits within 6 months. It is unclear how ECT works, but it is thought to affect neurotransmitter, peptide, and/or neuroendocrine functioning.

Light therapy has proven useful for depression which is seasonal in nature. Very bright lights for periods of 2-3 hours are usually effective within 2-4 days, but relapse occurs if the therapy is discontinued. Light therapy may affect circadian rhythms, which are presumed to be dysregulated; circadian rhythms also affect sleeping.

Psychological therapies have been proven effective only for unipolar depression, either alone or in conjunction with medication. Cognitive and cognitive-behavioral approaches are based on Beck's model and address the link between cognitions, emotion, and behavior. Collaborative empiricism involves the therapist and patient working together to identify, analyze, and test the validity of the patient's dysfunctional cognitions. Specific techniques for changing faulty beliefs and thought processes result in reductions in depressed mood. Behavioral strategies, such as scheduling pleasant events and concrete homework assignments, are also often used. Therapy outcome studies have supported the efficacy of cognitive therapy, which has been found to be more effective than minimal treatment and as effective as medication treatment.

Interpersonal psychotherapy (IPT) was developed by Weissman and Weissman and is based on a psychodynamic framework (i.e., disrupting bonds with a parent can initiate depression). IPT is more directive and time-limited than most psychodynamic treatments and addresses childhood, family background, and developmental issues only in terms of their relevance to current problems. Therapy focuses on helping patients identify the interpersonal conflicts in their lives, developing strategies for more successful communication and conflict negotiation, and coping more effectively with interpersonal stressors. Research has supported the efficacy of IPT in treating depression.

Marital therapy that emphasized increased feelings of closeness, open sharing of thoughts and feelings, positive interchanges, and effective problem solving for marital disputes was developed by Beach & O'Leary. This is effective in reducing depression and in improving marital satisfaction in depressed women. It has been recognized as an effective treatment for depression.

Comparative outcome research has examined the relative efficacy of treatments for depression. Both cognitive therapy and IPT have been found to be more effective than minimal treatment conditions, and IPT reduces the likelihood of relapse. NIMH conducted a comparative study of cognitive therapy, IPT, antidepressant medication, and placebos with 239 depressed persons. All patients showed improvement (see Figure 7.3 and Figure 7.4 on pages 229-230). More severely depressed patients benefited more from active medication compared to placebo, and IPT also showed significant improvement. Cognitive therapy was not statistically significantly superior to placebo. Criticisms of the study include differences in results based on the site, variations in type of cognitive therapy provided, the statistical analyses used, and the brief treatment provided. Follow-up data at 18 months showed only 24% had recovered and not relapsed; results suggests that cognitive therapy might help maintain improvement, but results were not statistically significant.

Combination treatments, which are consistent with the biopsychosocial approach, may have the following results: fewer patients may drop out of therapy, perhaps because it achieves a faster response than single treatments; the overall response rate over 3-4 months is not different from that of single treatments; and psychological treatment, either with or without medication, appears to be effective in preventing relapse or recurrence.

KEY IDEAS AND OBJECTIVES FOR STUDENTS

After reading the chapter, you should be able to answer each of the following questions:

1. What are the two major types of mood episodes? What are the two subtypes of these?

2. What are the major clusters of symptoms of a major depressive episode and what do these include?

3. What are the symptoms and characteristics of manic episodes? What are the characteristics and symptoms of hypomanic episodes?

4. What is the relationship between mood episodes and mood disorders? In other words, what are the different mood disorders and what kinds of mood disorders characterize each disorder

5. What are specifiers and how do they describe mood disorders?

6. What are the characteristics and symptoms of dysthymic and cyclothymic disorder?

7. What is the prevalence of major depression? How does prevalence vary by gender, age, income level, race/ethnicity?

8. What other disorders frequently occur in individuals with mood disorders? How does this affect treatment and recovery?

9. What is the relationship between depression and suicide?

10. How do gender, age, socioeconomic status, and race/ethnicity affect the rate of suicide attempts and completed suicides?

11. What are the warning signs of suicide and how can the risk of suicide be decreased?

12. What evidence is there from family, twin, and adoption studies to suggest a genetic basis to mood disorders? How are they transmitted?

13. What is the psychodynamic view of depression?

14. What is the cognitive perspective of depression?

15. How do interpersonal problems, especially social stressors, lack of social support and marital difficulties, contribute to the development and maintenance of depression? What is the emphasis of the interactional perspective?

16. What is the biopsychosocial perspective of mood disorders and is it supported by research?

17. What drug treatments, including tricyclic antidepressants, selective serotonin reuptake inhibitors (SSRIs) and monoamine oxidase inhibitors (MAOIs) are effective with bipolar depression? Which are effective with unipolar depression? What are their side effects?

18. How effective is electroconvulsive therapy (ECT) in the treatment of depression? Is it safe?

19. Is light therapy effective in treating mood disorders? Which disorders are appropriate for this treatment?

20. What is the focus of cognitive therapy of depression? Is it as effective as other treatments? How does it affect relapse?

21. What assumptions are the basis of marital therapy and interpersonal treatment for depression? What is the effectiveness of each?

22. Using the biopsychosocial approach, which treatment(s) should be used for mood disorders? How do medication and psychotherapy compare in their effectiveness?

Mood Disorders in the Movies

1. Mr. Jones (1993, Columbia TriStar, 114 min) The central character in this film presents with bipolar disorder. During a manic phase, the character exhibits pressured speech, grandiosity, flight of ideas, and impulsivity in the form of spending large sums of money, hypersexuality, and conducting the orchestra at a symphony performance. A depressive phase is also shown, and the link between creativity and bipolar disorder is demonstrated. Students can identify many of the symptoms of manic and depressive episodes. Inpatient treatment is provided when the character's functioning worsens.

Questions after watching the movie:

1. Given the text's description of the symptoms that are typical for an individual with a diagnosis of bipolar I disorder, how well did the movie do in presenting an accurate portrayal of this disorder? What "errors" (including errors of omission and commission) were made?

2. How did the film deal with the etiology of this disorder? What were the major consistencies (or inconsistencies) with contemporary theories?

3. How did the film deal with the issue of "treatment" or "cure?" What were the major consistencies (or inconsistencies) with contemporary theories?

4. If you were to be a consultant on a "remake" of this film, what advice would you give the director to help make the symptoms, etiology, and treatment more contemporary?

Using Case Studies in Abnormal Psychology by Meyer and Osborne:
The Affective Disorders and Suicide

General Summary

Chapter 7 of the casebook presents case material on mood disorders and suicide with specific information on Major Depressive Disorder with a suicide attempt, suicide, and Bipolar Disorder with Psychotic Features. By presenting the case of Joseph Westbecker, the chapter raises the controversy surrounding the drug, Prozac. The link between creativity and mental illness is also explored in the case of Virginia Woolf, which is a nice extension from the focus box presented in the text.

Case Comparisons

1. Major Depressive Disorder Associated with a Suicide Attempt: The Case of Joseph Westbecker. The initial diagnosis of Joseph was major depressive disorder. The diagnostic criteria for this disorder are summarized on page 192. Provide a summary of the specific characteristics of Joseph that initially supported the diagnosis using each of these criteria. Are any of the criteria questionable? What factors led to a change in Joseph's diagnosis? What factors may have led to the development of the problem for Joseph? Which theoretical models are linked to these factors? What treatment options were considered? Which was used?

2. Bipolar Disorder: The Case of Virginia Woolf. The diagnostic criteria for a manic episode are summarized on page 195 of the text. Provide a summary of the specific characteristics of Virginia that support the diagnosis using each of the criteria (be sure to include the symptoms of major depressive episode AND manic episodes). Are any of the criteria questionable? What factors may have led to the development of this problem for Virginia? Which theoretical models are linked to these factors? What treatment options were considered? Which treatments would be considered if she were alive today?

Integrating Perspectives
A Biopsychosocial Model

Use the Case of Joseph Westbecker to demonstrate the biopsychosocial model and the interactive effects of biological, psychological, and social factors.

Biological Factors

- Joseph's maternal grandmother was twice placed in a state mental hospital, reportedly showing depression, suicidal ideation, and delusions of persecution.
- Joseph's eating habits often consisted of cookies and ice cream (sometimes a gallon at a time) and often a dozen or more Diet Pepsi's a day.

Psychological Factors

- Joseph's father died just before his first birthday. His mother moved back in with her parents and her father was appointed Joseph's guardian. But, less than a year later, he was killed at his railroad job. Two years later, the only adult male figure in his life, his paternal grandfather, died of heart disease.

- Joseph was married twice and legally separated from his second wife (although he continued to have a relationship with her until his death). Relationships were always difficult.

Social Factors

- Joseph's family had many financial and emotional problems. He spent a year in an orphanage when he was 12-13. His family moved many times and his schooling was disrupted. He never obtained his GED which limited his employment opportunities.

Sample Multiple-Choice Questions

1. The two major types of mood episodes are ______ and ______.
   a. major depressive, hypomanic
   b. major depressive, manic
   c. cyclothymic, dysthymic
   d. manic, cyclothymic

2. Margarita is a 20 year-old college student who lives in the northern part of the country and finds that every year during the winter months, she becomes excessively fatigued, has a craving for carbohydrates, and puts on weight. As the spring approaches, Margarita notices that her symptoms disappear, even without specific treatment. Joanne is most likely suffering from _____.
   a. dysthymia
   b. cyclothymia
   c. bipolar disorder
   d. seasonal affective disorder

3. Lenora is a 45-year-old postal employee who was evaluated at a local mental health clinic. She claims to have felt constantly depressed for as long as she can remember, without really a period of "normal" mood for more than a few days at a time. Her depression has been accompanied by lethargy, little or no interest or pleasure in anything, trouble concentrating, and feelings of worthlessness. Her only periods of normal mood occur when she is home alone, watching TV or reading. Lenora is most likely suffering from _____.
   a. dysthymic depression
   b. manic depression
   c. bipolar depression
   d. cyclothymic depression

4. According to the focus box, Thinking about Gender Issues, several explanations have been offered to help account gender differences in depression. Which of the following possible explanations, proposed by Nolen-Hoeksema, has received strong support and appears to be very promising?
   a. The genetic hypothesis
   b. The hormonal hypothesis
   c. The artifact hypothesis
   d. The rumination hypothesis

5. Approximately _____ percent of individuals with a mood disorder eventually commit suicide.
   a. 15
   b. 30
   c. 45
   d. 70

6. Following the breakup of Alton's 10 year marriage, he became quite depressed. His depressive symptoms got so severe that Alton began having work-related difficulties, socially withdrew from virtually everyone, became highly self-critical, and lost what little self-esteem he had. Alton's therapist felt that his depression was the result of disturbances in close relationships (e.g., with his ex-wife and friends) and his poor self-esteem. Treatment focused on the interaction of personality factors, previous relationships, and the recent stress Alton had experienced. Alton's therapist is most likely using a _____ approach to therapy.
   a. cognitive
   b. psychoanalytic
   c. behavioral
   d. cognitive-behavioral

7. Leslie has been diagnosed with a mood disorder. Many times she finds that negative thoughts pop into her head and cause her a great deal of stress. Specifically, when her boyfriend does not compliment her on her appearance Leslie often says things like, "He didn't say he likes the way I look. He must hate me." Such automatic thoughts are examples of _____.
   a. arbitrary inferences
   b. overgeneralizations
   c. magnification
   d. minimization

8. The _____ theory hypothesizes that the needs and demands of people who are depressed place a strain on their interpersonal relationships.
   a. cognitive distortion
   b. hopelessness
   c. interactional
   d. diathesis-stress

9. According to the box, Integrating Perspectives: A Biopsychosocial Model, a person with too many stressors, failures, and poor interpersonal experiences may develop a negative schema. Which of the following is NOT included as part of a negative schema?
   a. Little hope that things will improve in the future
   b. Childhood, physical or life traumas
   c. Lack of confidence in ability to cope
   d. No expectations of support from others

10. Rusty has been suffering from depression for a number of years. His most notable symptoms aside from depressed mood, include mood reactivity, increased sleep and appetite, feeling weighted down or very heavy, and extreme sensitivity to interpersonal rejection. Which group of drugs used to treat depression appears to work BEST for Rusty's symptoms?
    a. Tricyclic antidepressants
    b. Selective serotonin reuptake inhibitors
    c. Monoamine oxidase inhibitors
    d. Anxiolytics

Answer Key

1. b
2. d
3. a
4. d
5. a
6. b
7. a
8. c
9. b
10. c

CHAPTER 8 SEXUAL DISORDERS

Sexual Dysfunction

The formal scientific study of sexual disorders began with the work of Richard von Krafft-Ebing, a professor at the University of Vienna. Dr. von Krafft-Ebbing is credited with having written the first text on the scientific analysis of sexual disorders. Sigmund Freud emphasized the importance of human sexuality in the study of clinical disorders and this continues to be a major emphasis of psychoanalysis.

In American, major contributions were made by Alfred Kinsey, and Masters and Johnson. Kinsey is most famous for his surveys of the sexual preferences and practices of American men and women. These surveys were published in 1948 and 1953 and are credited for paving the way for the objective observation of sexual activity. Masters and Johnson provided observational data on a variety of explicit sexual acts, such as masturbation, intercourse, and oral sex.

Sexual difficulties are common. It is estimated that as many as 36% of men have difficulties with premature ejaculation and 16% have difficulty obtaining or maintaining erections at some point in their life. The DSM-IV identifies four major categories of sexual dysfunction: Desire disorders, arousal disorders, orgasmic disorders, and pain disorders. Desire refers to how often or strongly a person wants sex, arousal to how excited someone becomes once sex is initiated, and orgasm to the male's ability to ejaculate and the female's capacity to reach climax after arousal. Sexual dysfunction is diagnosed only if it is not the result of some other disorder, such as major depression.

Desire Disorders

Description. The two major sexual desire disorders are hypoactive sexual desire (HSD) and sexual aversion disorder. HSD is marked by the absence of sexual fantasies and the wish for sexual activity. Sexual aversion disorder involves avoiding all or almost all genital sexual contact with a partner and causes definite personal or interpersonal distress.

Causes. Sexual desire seems linked to hormones. In particular the level of testosterone seems linked to HSD. Individuals with HSD have been found to have lower levels of testosterone than individuals not meeting criteria for HSD.

Depression and severe stress may also cause HSD. While the person's sexual desire typically returns when the depression lifts or stressful life circumstances change, for some the condition persists. Individuals with HSD have higher rates of lifetime depression than individuals not meeting criteria for HSD.

Child sexual abuse and rape have also been linked to desire disorders. Sexual problems seem to be caused by or become enmeshed with feelings of anxiety, anger, jealousy, and guilt. Such feelings have been hypothesized to be the result of unconscious conflicts that are expressed by the individual selectively focusing on the negative characteristics of their partners or situations.

Interpersonal problems often cause sexual disorders.

Arousal Disorders

Description. Male erectile disorder is the persistent or recurrent failure to attain or maintain an adequate erection until completion of sexual activity. The man with lifelong erectile disorder has never been able to have intercourse with a partner. In acquired erectile disorder, the man is currently unable to achieve a sufficient erection to engage in sexual intercourse but was able to do so at least once in the past. Female sexual arousal disorder is characterized by a woman's persistent or recurrent failure to be physiologically aroused until completion of sexual activity. As with males, this may be a lifelong or acquired problem.

Causes. Male erectile disorder was once thought to be primarily the result of psychological factors. Today, it is estimated that more than 50% of all cases have organic causes. The presence of drugs, such as antidepressants, increase erectile problems. Aging is linked to increased problems with obtaining or maintaining an erection. Organic causes are often diagnosed by measuring nocturnal penile tumescence (NPT). Since most men experience an average of about 1 erection every 90 while sleeping, NPT can confirm organic causes of male erectile disorder. Many cases of erectile disorder involve both organic and psychological causes, and psychological treatment is often effective, despite some degree of physical impairment.

Psychological causes are divided into (a) historical influences and (b) those currently maintaining the sexual problem. Rigid adherence to orthodox religious beliefs and practices is a common factor in the backgrounds of men and women with different forms of sexual dysfunction. Other historical influences include: having a dominating, overcontrolling parent, having a traumatic initial sexual encounter, or experiencing homosexual leanings. Anxiety is seen as the most important current factor regardless of the historical cause of the sexual disorder. Performance anxiety leads to a feeling Masters and Johnson call spectatoring. That is, the man grows self-conscious and becomes an observer of his sexual response looking for signs of failure.

Much less is know about the causes of female sexual arousal disorder. For the female, the clitoris is the organ that is sensitive to sexual stimulation. Anything that reduces the flow of oxygen-rich blood to it may impair sexual arousal and orgasm.

Orgasmic Disorders

Description. Orgasmic disorders, including female orgasmic disorder and male orgasmic disorder, are characterized by the persistent or recurrent delay in or absence of orgasm following adequate sexual arousal. As with arousal disorders, these are divided into three subtypes based on whether they are (a) lifelong or acquired, (b) generalized or confined to a specific situation, or (c) due primarily to psychological or combined psychological and medical factors.

Causes. For men, the most common causes of orgasmic disorders are restrictive religious prohibitions, homosexual commitments, and negative family influences. For women, emotional dissatisfaction with her partner is the most common cause. Sexual problems in women can also result from experiencing specific traumas (such as rape), being molested as a child, or feeling severe pain or panic during the first sexual encounter. Masters and Johnson concluded that most forms of sexual dysfunction in women are rooted in society's double-standard of sexual values: Male sexuality is culturally sanctions, if not implicitly encouraged, while women's sexual nature has been ignored, even denied. This issue is discussed in detail on page 246 in the "Thinking about Social Issues" box.

Premature ejaculation occurs when the male ejaculates too soon. It is difficult to define "too soon," but the DSM-IV suggests "minimal sexual stimulation before, on, or shortly after penetration and before the person wishes it" is premature ejaculation. Masters and Johnson report that better educated men who are concerned with their ability to satisfy their partners are most likely to complain about premature ejaculation. Men who did not complete high school rarely complained.

Pain Disorders

Women who experience dyspareunia, or painful intercourse, often lack adequate vaginal lubrication. Emotional or interpersonal factors are usually responsible for this problem. However, physical factors such as vaginal infections that damage the ligaments supporting the uterus may be the cause.

Vaginismus refers to involuntary tightening in the outer one-third of the vagina. These spasms make it difficult, if not impossible, for the woman to have intercourse.

Treatment of Male Sexual Dysfunction

Psychological Therapies. Current psychological treatment methods of male sexual dysfunction are largely derived from Masters and Johnson's sex therapy. The core assumption of this therapy is that sexual dysfunction stems mainly from the fear of failure to perform. The following key concepts for the basis of the typical therapy program:

1. Desensitization. Decrease pressure to perform by requiring that the couple not engage in sexual intercourse, but to begin a carefully graduated program of mutually pleasurable sensual and sexual involvement. The program is self-paced with no explicit goals to undercut all performance anxiety.

2. Sensate focus is emphasized. This procedure involves the mutual, non-goal oriented sensual interaction between partners which involves physical stimulation of each other's body. The couple is taught to give and receive pleasure, first through nongenital contact and then, by

specific genital stimulation. This process increases verbal and nonverbal communication and teaches the couple that sexual gratification does not necessarily depend on intercourse.

3. Focus on couples. Both partners are part of the treatment, even if only one is identified as having a problem.

Surgical and Pharmacological Treatments. Men with erectile disorders can receive a penile implant which involves the insertion of a semirigid rod or hydraulic device that can be pumped up to produce an erection. While most men who receive implants report that they would choose the surgery again, if confronted with the same problem, 25% are significantly dissatisfied with the outcome. Dissatisfaction focused on the size and stiffness of their erections and decreased sensations during ejaculation.

Drugs, such as papaverine or phentolamine, have been used to produce partially or completely stiff erections that last 1 to 4 hours. Follow-up studies indicate that men who use drugs to produce erections report that the vast majority of the men experience satisfactory erections. They inject themselves approximately 5 times per month and report more frequent orgasm, greater sexual satisfaction, less depression and anxiety, and enhanced self-esteem. Negative effects include scarring of the penis, liver problems, and occasional experiences of prolonged erection in the absence of sexual stimulation.

Treatment of Female Sexual Dysfunction

Many of the basic treatment concepts and procedures described for dysfunctional men are appropriate for dysfunctional women. In particular, procedures such as sensate focus exercises encourage the woman to show her partner what she does and does not find sexually arousing.

Several additional treatment procedures have proved effective in enhancing female sexual responsiveness. Once such procedure is a systematic program of directed masturbation. The woman is taught to familiarize herself with her body, particularly the genital area, and to identify pleasurable sensations. A female therapist then instructs the woman in the intricacies of masturbation, including the use of electric vibrators. Once the woman reaches orgasm through masturbation, her partner is introduced to the procedure by observing her masturbate. Next he learns to use masturbate her to orgasm.

Summarizing Treatment Effectiveness

Most sexual disorders require a multimodal treatment approach, including many components: education, desensitization of performance anxiety, changing negative attitudes and dysfunctional beliefs about sex, and improving communication between partners. Combinations of psychological and medical treatment are often required.

Paraphilias

Description

Paraphilias are sexual disorders in which bizarre or unusual acts, imagery, or objects are required for sexual stimulation. Many factors have limited our ability to accurately identify and describe this population. Research from Abel and his colleagues suggest that (a) the average paraphiliac commits many other crimes, (b) they engage in as many as 10 different forms of paraphilia, and (c) they often have normal sexual involvement with adult partners that do not involve paraphiliac fantasies or activities.

Exhibitionism. This individual exposes his genitals to unsuspecting individuals or has strong and persistent urges and sexually arousing fantasies concerning such exposure. The focus box on page 255 (Thinking about Controversial Issues) provides a present day example of exhibitionism, Pee Wee Herman and the controversy surrounding what constitutes true "exhibitionism."

Voyeurism. The voyeur is a male whose preferred or exclusive means of gaining sexual excitement is observing unsuspecting women undressing or engaging in sexual activity.

Masochism and Sadism. The masochist is sexually aroused by fantasizing about or engaging in the act of being dominated, humiliated, or even beaten. The sadist is aroused by fantasies or actions involving the domination or beating of another person.

Fetishism. This disorder involves becoming sexually aroused by persistent fantasies about or actual use of nonliving objects, such as women's panties.

Transvestic Fetishism. A transvestite is a man who becomes sexually aroused by dressing as a woman. Often this is done with the knowledge of and occasionally the cooperation of his wife. For the most part, these men are masculine in appearance and activities. Most are heterosexual and married.

Pedophilia involves the unnatural desire to have sexual contact with a prepubescent child. The contact may vary from genital contact to sexual intercourse. While the alarming incidence of child sexual abuse may appear to be a recent phenomenon, the problem was first identified some 100 years ago by Sigmund Freud. Virtually all of his female patients who suffered from what Freud called "hysterical illness" reported having been sexually abused as children. Freud hypothesized that child sexual abuse was the main cause of adult neurotic behavior. This idea called the seduction theory of neurosis was widely rejected by Freud's colleges. Freud decided that his patients had not really experienced incest, rather, they had unconsciously wished to have sex with their fathers. This new theory was called the theory of infantile sexuality and became the cornerstone of psychoanalysis.

Other Paraphilias include (a) frotteurism, sexual urges involving touching or rubbing against a nonconsenting and unsuspecting person, (b) necrophilia, sexual obsession with corpses, perhaps including intercourse, (c) klismaphilia, sexual excitement that results from having enemas, (d) coprophilia, sexual interest in feces, and (e) zoophilia, sexual gratification from having sexual activity with animals.

Causes

Psychodynamic Theory. According to this theory, all paraphilias are expressions of a common underlying psychopathology related to unconscious intrapsychic conflicts originating in early childhood. Prominent psychoanalysts argue that sexual aggression is simply an extreme form of the same sexual drive that arouses people who engage in conventional sexual activities. Abel rejects this theory pointing to evidence that shows that paraphiliacs suffer from a generalized lack of control over their sexual arousal and behavior.

Cognitive-Behavioral Theory. This theory focuses on the role of learning in the development of paraphilias. Masturbation may be the key is that young men masturbate frequently and early in their psychological development. When they do, they fantasize about a variety of specific sexual stimuli, sometimes deviant or unconventional. Likewise, parents may model and maintain deviant sexuality patterns through direct and vicarious reinforcement.

A Psychobiological Model. John Money and Margaret Lamacz have proposed a theory of the early development of paraphilias that focus on the complex links between anatomy, hormones, and life experiences. During the ages of 5 and 8 years, a lovemap is developed which determines what sexual imagery and actions an individual will find stimulating. Traumatic childhood experiences, such as sexual abuse, can have a disruptive influence on the development of the lovemap. Errors may become programmed into the map that involve either the displacement or distortion of elements within the sequence of behaviors that normally lead to sexual activity for that species. Thus, fondling a sexual partner (which is normal for humans) may be replaced by rubbing against an unsuspecting stranger. These authors believe that having a strict upbringing puts individuals at risk for the development of paraphilias.

Treatment

Psychological Treatments. Lengthy psychodynamic therapies have not proven effective with these problems, but alternative therapies (cognitive-behavioral and drug therapies) have been successful. Cognitive-behavioral treatments focus on five major areas: (1) suppression or elimination of the individual's unwanted or undesirable sexual arousal; (2) substitution of a more acceptable source of sexual arousal and behavior; (3) development of self-control or coping skills to resist the problem behavior; (4) cognitive restructuring; (5) relapse prevention training.

Covert sensitization is a common treatment strategy for suppression of unwanted sexual arousal. This technique involves the use of imagery that links a negative consequence with the unwanted activity. Orgasmic reconditioning appears helpful to change paraphiliac develop sexual arousal to more conventional heterosexual activities. Self-control strategies help the person to learn to recognize early warning signs of temptation. Social-skills training helps the individual learn how to relate better to adult partners. Cognitive restructuring helps alter distorted thinking. Finally, relapse prevention training prepares patients to cope with threats to self-control and thus to prevent relapse.

Pharmacological therapies. Hormonal agents (such as Cyproterone acetate, an antiandrogen drug, have been found to virtually eliminate relapse among paraphiliacs when used in high doses. The antidepressant drug, Prozac, has been shown to significantly decrease deviant fantasies and behavior without interfering with conventional heterosexual functioning.

Gender Identity Disorders

Gender-Identity Disorder

Description. Gender-role identity is the individual's perception of himself or herself as consistently male or female. Individuals with gender-identity disorder want to be members of the opposite sex. Before the development of the DSM-IV, this disorder was called transsexual.

Causes. Prenatal hormones have been suggested as a possible cause of gender-identity disorder. Both psychodynamic and behavioral theories emphasize the importance of early childhood experiences. Psychodynamic theories believe that for normal sexual development to occur, the child must identify successfully with the parent of the opposite sex. Behavioral theorists also focus on parents as role models and sources of social reinforcement. Despite these theories, researchers cannot predict with any certainty which children will develop gender-identity disorders or which will become transsexual as adults.

Treatment. Sex reassignment surgery is an established form of treating transsexuals. In male-to-female reassignment, the man takes estrogen to develop breasts and other female characteristics. He is then castrated and an artificial clitoris and vagina are constructed. In the female-to-male reassignment, the woman initially takes androgens to reduce her breasts, develop male characteristics, and stop menstruation. Her uterus and remaining breast tissue is removed and a penis is constructed. The effectiveness of surgical procedures is modest. The best estimate is that roughly two-thirds of patients show improved adjustment following surgery.

Psychological treatment has been limited primarily to behavioral methods, though controlled studies are lacking and few therapists have adopted these methods.

Sexual Disorders Not Otherwise Specified

One example of a disorder in this category is 'Persistent and Marked Distress about Sexual Orientation." This category is linked to one of the most controversial aspects of abnormal psychology. In the second edition of the DSM, homosexuality was listed as a major clinical disorder. In the third edition, this was removed. While the word, homosexuality cannot be found in the DSM IV, this category seems to refer to anxiety over being homosexual, not heterosexual.

Psychodynamic theory was very influential in shaping clinicians' views of homosexuality. In this model, homosexuality is the result of having an overprotective, close-binding mother and is seen as fixation at an immature level of psychosexual development.

Several major research finding in the past few years have established the biological basis of homosexuality. These studies show that (a) brains of homosexual and heterosexual individuals differ, (b) twin studies and DNA patterning show high concordance rates between individuals identified as homosexual and family members, and (c) gay and heterosexual men differ in cognitive abilities that reflect differences in brain architecture.

It should be obvious that the implication of this biological model is that changing an adult's sexual orientation should be difficult, if not impossible. In stead of trying to change sexual orientation, current therapies are designed to help gays and lesbians lead more fulfilling lives as homosexuals.

KEY IDEAS AND OBJECTIVES FOR STUDENTS

After reading the chapter, you should be able to answer each of the following questions:

1. What are the major divisions of sexual dysfunction?

2. What are the biological causes of sexual dysfunctions?

3. What are the psychological causes of sexual dysfunctions?

4. From what methods does modern sex therapy stem?

5. For what problems are surgical and pharmacological treatments useful?

6. What are paraphilias?

7. What are the primary types of paraphilias?

8. What are the characteristics of people with gender-identity disorder (formerly known as transsexualism)?

9. What are the characteristics of 'Sexual Disorders Not Otherwise Specified, under the category of dissatisfaction with sexual orientation? Does this include all homosexual individuals?

Sexual Dysfunction and Sexual Disorders in the Movies

Sadism and Masochism. The film, Exit to Eden, (1994, HBO Video, 113 min) provides a view of the world of Paraphilia. The island is a resort where individuals with sadistic and masochistic tendencies can openly "satisfy" their erotic fantasies. The film is a comedy, but several scenes provide a perspective on the role of early experiences in the development of paraphilias.

Questions after watching the movie.

1. What examples of Masochism, Sadism, and Fetishism were presented in the film? Why are these activities considered atypical for our culture?

2. Which characters in the film perceived these activities to be a sign of a problem? Which did not?

Tranvestic Fetishism vs. Gender Identity Disorder. Several films have focused on the Crossdressing. These include: Tootsie (1982, Columbia TriStar, 116 min), Victor/Victoria (1982, MGA/UA, 134 min), Mrs. Doubtfire (1993, Fox Video, 120 min), and the recent To Wong Foo, Thanks for Everything, Julie Newmar (1995, MCA/Universial, 108 min). While each film shows individuals who decide to disguise themselves as someone of the opposite sex and to cross dress, not all of these individuals would receive a diagnosis of Transvestic Fetishism or Gender Identity Disorder.

Questions after watching the movie.

1. Which characters in these movies could receive a diagnosis of Transvestic Fetishism? Gender Identity Disorder (Transsexualism)?

2. Should we treat these disorders? If so, what should treatment emphasize?

Using Case Studies in Abnormal Behavior by Meyer and Osborne:
Dissociative Disorders

General Summary

Chapter 3 presents case material for several sexual disorders including paraphilias, transvestism, impotence, and female sexual dysfunction.

Case Comparisons

Paraphilias: The Case of Jeffrey Dahmer. The diagnostic criteria for paraphilias are presented on pages 252 - 258 of the text. As the authors note, the case of Jeffrey Dahmer does not fit into one clear type of paraphilia, but seems to be a mixture of several. What specific characteristics of Dahmer support the diagnosis of paraphilia. What type(s) of paraphilias did he have? What factors may have led to the development of this problem for Dahmer? Which theoretical models are linked to these factors? What treatment options were used?

Male Erectile Disorder (Male Sexual Dysfunction): The Case of Tim. The diagnostic criteria for male erectile disorder are summarized on page 239 of the text. Provide a summary of the specific characteristics of Tim's case that support the diagnosis using each of the three criteria. Are any of the criteria questionable? What factors may have led to the development of this problem for Tim? Which theoretical models are linked to these factors? What treatment options were considered? Which was used?

Female Sexual Arousal Disorder (Female Psychosexual Dysfunction): The Case of Virginia. The diagnostic criteria for female sexual arousal disorder are summarized on page 239 of the text. Provide a summary of the specific characteristics of Virginia's case that support the diagnosis using each of the three criteria. Are any of the criteria questionable? What factors may have led to the development of this problem for Virginia? Which theoretical models are linked to these factors? What treatment options were considered? Which was used?

Integrating Perspectives
A Biopsychosocial Model

The Case of Virginia: Perspectives on Female Sexual Arousal Disorder

Biological Factors

•Virginia had a physical disorder, vaginismus, which contributed to her arousal problems.
•Three months before she was married, she developed a vaginal infection that sensitized her concerns with sexually transmitted diseases.

Psychological Factors

•Learning apparently played a large role in Virginia's problems. Not only did she feel that sex was sinful, but more importantly, she felt that it was shameful and dirty.
•Virginia rejected many of her normal bodily sensations and saw these as cues for anxiety. Although she was able to masturbate to orgasm, she experienced much guil t in the process.
•Her husband's inexperience made their first attempt at intercourse cumbersome and unsatisfying.

Social Factors

•Religion played a role in Virginia's problems. She was taught early that the expression of sexuality outside of marriage was wrong and she began to experience guilt and anxiety, particularly when she began to masturbate at age 16.
•Virginia's experience with the insensitive gynecologist also played a role in her problem. Many physicians have little training in how to deal with these types of problems. His rough examination combined with a poor bedside manner helped keep her from seeking out appropriate medical treatment.

Sample Multiple-Choice Questions

1. Joe derives a great deal of sexual satisfaction by rubbing against unsuspecting women on the subway. Joe is engaging in _______.
   a. frotteurism
   b. exhibitionism
   c. voyeurism
   d. sadism

2. John is beginning to think something is wrong with him. He never fantasizes about sex and he never wants to have sex with his wife. It is likely that John has _______ disorder.
   a. sexual aversion
   b. male sexual desire
   c. hypoactive sexual desire
   d. male erectile

3. George is very self-conscious during sexual activities. During sexual activity George often observes his sexual responses and looks for any sign that he is a failure when it comes to sex. This is called _______.
   a. aversive conditioning
   b. expectation of sexual failure
   c. approach avoidance
   d. spectatoring

4. On Friday night Tom went to a party with his wife, Jill. Tom consumed six beers at the party and later that night tried to have sex with Jill. Tom was unable to get an erection. The next night Tom tried to have sex with Jill, but he was really anxious about whether or not he could obtain an erection and Jill kept pressuring him to have sex with her. The _______ perspective best explains Tom's erectile failures.
   a. psychological
   b. multidetermined
   c. biological
   d. biopsychosocial

5. Tina prefers oral sex to vaginal intercourse because vaginal intercourse causes Tina to feel painful burning and itching sensations. Tina is most likely suffering from _______.
   a. vaginismus
   b. female sexual pain disorder
   c. dyspareunia
   d. female sexual arousal disorder

6. The main problem with the information available about paraphilias is that _______.
   a. it was mostly obtained through observational methods
   b. it was mostly obtained from chronic drug users
   c. it was mostly obtained from men who have been imprisoned for their deviant sexual behavior
   d. it was mostly obtained from men who were in court ordered therapy for their deviant sexual behavior

7. Joe derives a great deal of sexual satisfaction by looking into unsuspecting women's bedroom windows and watching them undress. He usually masturbates while watching these women undress. Tom's disorder is called _______.
   a. exhibitionism
   b. fetishism
   c. frotteurism
   d. voyeurism

8. Roger becomes sexually aroused when he wears make-up and a dress with pantyhose and high heels. Roger's disorder is called _______.
   a. homosexual fetishism
   b. transvestic fetishism
   c. transsexual fetishism
   d. bisexual fetishism

9. Tim was seeing a therapist for treatment of masochism. This therapist had Tim masturbate to his usual masochistic fantasies, but just before climax Tim was instructed to switch to a conventional heterosexual erotic fantasy. Tim was being treated with _______.
   a. covert sensitization
   b. aversive conditioning
   c. cognitive restructuring
   d. orgasmic reconditioning

10. Jeff, a homosexual, goes to see a therapist because he wants to know what caused him to be homosexual. Jeff's therapist tells him that his homosexuality is the result of having an over-protective mother and an insensitive, cold father. Jeff's therapist adheres to the _______ theory.
   a. psychodynamic
   b. behavioral
   c. cognitive
   d. cognitive-behavioral

Answer Key

1. a
2. c
3. d
4. d
5. c
6. c
7. d
8. b
9. d
10. a

CHAPTER 9 SUBSTANCE-RELATED DISORDERS

The Hebrew Bible, written 2,500 years ago, describes the essential features of alcoholism including physical and psychological dependence, alcohol induced memory deficits, and withdrawal. The authors of the Old and New Testaments warn against drunkenness, link it with sinful behavior, and severely admonish those who lack the strength to resist the temptation to imbibe. Consistent with these views of substance abuse, chronic alcohol abusers were killed and tortured through the Middle Ages and frequently confined to prison since they had chosen to engage in sinful behavior.

In the mid-eighteenth century a radical view developed that suggested alcoholism was a disease rather than sin. By the nineteenth century many physicians concluded that habitual use of drugs like the opiates, tobacco, and coffee stemmed from inherited or acquired biological vulnerability.

The worldwide temperance movement, which peaked at the beginning of the twentieth century, viewed alcohol as the cause of alcoholism. The movement advocated the control and prohibition of the sale of alcoholic products. Prohibition became law in the United States in 1919, shortly after the end of World War I. Prohibition was repealed in 1933.

Over the past 40 or 50 years, a more enlightened view of alcohol and drug abuse has emerged. A self-help group called Alcoholics Anonymous (AA) persuaded many Americans that alcoholism is more a medical and social problem than a moral one.

Until relatively recently, alcohol was the principal drug of abuse in Western society. Opium had been used in the Middle East, India and China, but until the eighteenth century, most Western opium addicts were either survivors of battlefield trauma or victims of chronic pain who had used opium, morphine, and heroin for their pain-killing properties. These drugs were not regulated until the Pure Food and Drug Act and the Harrison Narcotic Act were passed in the early twentieth century.

The abuse of drugs other than alcohol and the opiates in Western countries increased sharply in the early nineteenth century. This increase has been linked to (1) veterans of Napoleon's Egyptian campaign who brought back marijuana and hashish to France and (2) the introduction of cocaine, the potent alkaloid of the coca leaf, in the United States. Sigmund Freud and Sherlock Holmes promoted and popularized cocaine as a mental stimulant with magical analgesic and sedative properties with virtually no harmful consequences. Thus by the end of the nineteenth century, alcohol had become only one of the drugs that Americans abused.

Diagnosis Of Substance-Related Disorders

Alcohol and drug addictions were included in both DSM-I and DSM-II as varieties of sociopathic personality disturbance, a catchall diagnostic category that included antisocial behavior and the sexual disorders. The implication of this classification was that people diagnosed with these problems threatened society's moral fabric as a result of their intemperate or immoral behavioral choices.

The DSM-III gave the alcohol- and drug-related disorders their own separate category, the substance-use disorders. This classification eliminated the moralistic stigma of the previous manuals and highlighted new research findings that pointed to sociocultural and genetic factors in the etiology of these conditions. The DSM-III also established separate diagnoses for substance abuse and substance dependence.

DSM-IV evaluated the criteria from the DSM-III and DSM-III-R for substance abuse and dependence. DSM-IV reaffirmed the diagnostic emphasis on tolerance and withdrawal symptoms as critical factors for differentiating substance dependence from substance abuse. In the DSM-III, the diagnosis of substance dependence required the presence of either tolerance or withdrawal (or both) based on the assumption that dependence cannot develop in the absence of these symptoms. The drafters of the DSM-III-R concluded that a person could be dependent without demonstrating either symptoms. The DSM-IV work group, thought that the presence of these symptoms was important enough to distinguish between two types of addicted persons: Those with tolerance or withdrawal (diagnosed as with physiological dependence) and those without either symptoms (diagnosed as without physioloigcal dependence).

Tolerance occurs at both the cellular and the psychological levels. Cells adjust to the long-term presence of drugs in the bloodstream by altering certain biochemical processes to achieve physiological balance with the substances. Tolerance requires the individual to use more of the substance to maintain its original reinforcing effects.

Withdrawal refers to the physical and psychological symptoms that occur when the individual stops drug or alcohol intake after a period of use long enough to induce dependence. Symptoms include nausea, vomiting, restlessness and agitation, and sleeplessness.

Americans with Substance-Related Disorders

Between 5 and 7 percent of the U.S. population (14 to 16 million people) meet the DSM-IV criteria for alcohol abuse or dependence. Between 4 and 6 million Americans abuse illicit drugs. More than 45 million Americans are dependent on nicotine in cigarettes.

Rates of abuse and dependence vary with age, sex, and ethnicity. Men between the ages of 18 and 44 have rates more than double the overall rates. At most ages, African Americans and Hispanics of both sexes demonstrate slightly higher rates of abuse and dependence than whites.

Today, polysubstance abuse is more the rule than the exception. Most often this involves using alcohol and one or more additional substances. This trend is making it more difficult to get an accurate picture of the numbers of drug abusers in the United States.

The Nature and Cause of Substance Abuse

Alcohol Abuse and Dependence

In moderate doses, alcoholic beverages initially produce a mild sense of stimulation and enhanced well-being, followed by relaxation and calm. In larger doses, alcohol interferes with cognitive functioning, balance and coordination, judgment, memory, and perception. The amount of alcohol in the bloodstream is called the blood-alcohol level. High blood-alcohol levels are associated with risk of having an automobile accident, crime of all kinds, high risk sexual behavior, and increased levels of family violence.

In terms of health, chronic alcohol abuse is associated with permanent, disabling changes in brain function; birth defects, physical disorders affecting the brain, heart, liver, and gastrointestinal system. Chronic alcohol abuse is a major cause of premature death in the United States.

Nicotine Dependence

Tobacco contains nicotine, a substance that induces dependence. Nicotine is found in all forms of tobacco. The use of smokeless tobacco has increased in recent years, especially among young males. In contrast cigarette smoking has declined markedly in the United States since 1964, however, the decline in cigarette use has been very uneven among young people. Among high school seniors, whites are most likely and blacks least likely to be heavy smokers and drinkers. Rates for Hispanic youths fall in between.

Nicotine is a central nervous system stimulant that's chemically related to amphetamines. Nicotine causes withdrawal symptoms and tolerance and induces dependence. In low doses, nicotine acts as a mild CNS stimulant. At higher doses, it can cause agitation and irritability, interfere with thinking and problems solving, and bring on dramatic alterations in mood.

While the health hazards caused by cigarette smoking have been know for years, cigarette manufactures continue to deny that their products bring serious harm. This is discussed in detail in the "Thinking about Social Issues" focus box highlights the problems that the tobacco industry has had to face in defending their products.

Amphetamine Abuse and Dependence

Like nicotine, amphetamines are CNS stimulants. Methamphetamine, commonly called "speed," is the best-known and most commonly used member of this drug class. For many years, amphetamines were used to control appetite, reduce fatigue, and heighten concentration. These uses are no longer encouraged due to the drugs' abuse potential. One drug from this class, Ritalin, is still widely used to control the agitated behavior of children with attention-deficit hyperactivity disorder. Ritalin calms many of these children, even though it's a stimulant for adults.

Low to moderate doses of a stimulant lead to elevated mood and increased mental alertness and energy. In higher doses, stimulants produce hyperactivity and restlessness, insomnia, anxiety, impaired judgment, and even anger and fighting. Stimulant intoxication produces profound changes heartrate, blood pressure, gastrointestinal functioning, and respiration. Chronic use may result in emotional blunting (apathy), fatigue, sadness, and social withdrawal. Agitation, concentration difficulties, and paranoid delusions can occur upon taking increasing doses of these drugs repeatedly for an extended period of time.

Stimulant withdrawal typically involves a "crash": a period of profound despair and depression which can last for several days or more. Tolerance develops to the stimulants ability to produce euphoria and energy, thus, explaining why high doses of the drug are often taken.

Cocaine and "Crack" Abuse and Dependence

Cocaine is a short-acting, powerful stimulant which has effects similar to those of amphetamines, only shorter lived and more intense. When taken by mouth, cocaine's potency is significantly reduced. As a result it is generally inhaled ("snorted"), smoked, or injected. Crack is the dried mixture of the powdered hydrochloride salt of cocaine, water, and baking soda. It's smoked to yield a very intense, 20- to 30-minute "high."

Cocaine and crack cause dependence rapidly for two reasons: (1) the euphoria they produce is profoundly reinforcing and (2) the effect is so short lived and so often followed by depression that the abuser ingests repeated doses in an attempt to regain the high and postpone the low.

Sedative-Hypnotic Abuse and Dependence

The sedative-hypnotic drugs reduce brain activity, especially the activity of the reticular activating system (RAS). As a result, these drugs are commonly used to sedate and calm (in low doses) and to induce sleep (in higher doses). These drugs include the barbiturates, the benzodiazepines, the carbamates, and the barbiturate-like hypnotics.

The abuse potential of these drugs is very high. In low doses, they induce mild sedation, relaxation, and a sense of well-being. Higher doses induce behavioral and CNS depression and respiratory failure. Because these drugs produce profound tolerance, stopping use abruptly can cause a variety of life-threatening consequences, including convulsions, coma, and death.

Opioid Abuse and Dependence

Three groups are included in this drug class: (1) the natural opiates, morphine and codeine, (2) the semisynthetic opiates, heroin, and (3) the synthetic opiates, methadone, Darvon, and Demerol. Opiates produce euphoria and a profound sense of well-being, passivity, and warmth. The individual experiences a subjective sense of being removed from physical reality and put into a dreamlike state.

Both the natural and synthetic opiates are profoundly addicting. They induce rapid tolerance, physical dependence, and a disagreeable period of physical withdrawal that is characterized by nausea, vomiting, psychomotor irritability, and insomnia.

Hallucinogen Abuse and Dependence

The halucinogens include LSD, psilocybin, morning glory seeds, mescaline, and PCP. They are ingested to produce hallucinations. Reaching this altered state of consciousness is reinforcing to some people. Hallucinogens also have the potential to permanently alter neurotransmitter functioning in the brain and cause prolonged paranoid and delusional psychoses that are difficult to treat.

Cannabis (Marijuana and Hashish) Abuse and Dependence

Cannabis is related to the hallucinogens. The psychoactive ingredient in cannabis is tetrahydrocannabinol THC. In sufficient amounts, both marijuana and hashish can induce hallucinations and paranoid delusions. In moderate doses, individuals experience subjective effects such as a sense of relaxation and well-being. On occasion, individuals become disinhibited. Moderate doses of marijuana produce behavioral effects similar to those of moderate doses of alcohol.

The most troubling consequence of chronic use of marijuana is called the amotivational syndrome. This is characterized by the individual having great difficulty rousing himself from profound self-absorption to become reinvolved with friends, work, family, and school.

Causes of Substance Abuse and Dependence

Genetic/Biological Factors

Evidence for a biological cause of substance abuse and dependence comes from several sources. First, twin studies have confirmed the expected genetic relationship for alcoholism by showing a higher concordance rate for identical twins than for fraternal twins.

Second, adoption studies have shown that (1) sons of alcoholics are four times more likely than sons of nonalcoholics to become alcoholic adults, regardless of whether they had ben raised by their alcoholic biological parents or nonalcoholic adoptive parents, and (2) the influence of genetics on the daughters of alcoholics is not as strong as that for sons of alcoholics. Third, results reported from adoption studies looking at the incidence of drug abuse and cigarette smoking provide similar data to those with alcohol with the exception that sex differences have not been found.

Fourth, evoked potential (EP), a measure of the brain's electrical response to external stimuli, and event-related potential (ERP), a measure of electrical events that arise during the brain's processing of information, have been employed to study genetic influences on alcoholism. Sons of alcoholics show significant differences in a specific ERP response, P300, that is similar to that seen in chronic alcoholics who are not longer drinking.

In general, research does not support the idea that children of alcoholics and drug addicts are doomed to follow in their parents' footsteps. These children may bear "extra burdens in life" (as reviewed in the *Thinking about Research* focus box). Most researchers and clinicians believe that there is a heightened predisposition to developing the disorder based on biological and genetic factors.

Sociocultural Factors

Research has indicated that group membership (ethnic, religious, and national origin) plays a great role in alcohol consumption and the incidence of alcoholism. For example, New England has typically had the highest per capita consumption of alcohol in the US. The region is populated with large numbers of Northern Europeans, whose parents and grandparents came from countries with high alcoholism rates. Per capital consumption in this region is much higher than in the three southern census regions, which are populated with a substantial number of Southern Baptists, for whom drinking is forbidden.

The relationship between alcoholism and abstinence is not linear. That is, there are groups for who alcoholism is quite low, yet abstinence is also low (Italian Americans, Jewish Americans, and Chinese Americans). The opposite is also true: High rates of alcoholism and abstinence characterize Americans with Irish, African, and Eastern European heritage. In general, it appears that cultural groups that stress the moderate use of alcohol, especially in a family or religious context, produce large numbers of members who use alcohol but few alcoholics. Consequently, cultural groups that focus on both the dangers and the pleasures of alcohol use tend to produce more members who abstain from alcohol as well as more who drink to excess.

Gender differences have been shown to exist in the US, Canada, Puerto Rico, South Korea, and Taiwan. Overall, around 29 percent of men and only 4 percent of women can be diagnosed as being alcoholic at some point in their lives. Two theories have been proposed to account for this. First, most cultures have low tolerance for heavy alcohol use in women due to their traditional role in caring for children. Second, women appear to have a smaller amount of an enzyme necessary to detoxify alcohol in the stomach and small intestine. This would explain why alcohol consumed in equivalent doses by men and women has greater behavioral and physiological effects on women.

Learning-Based Factors

The conditioned compensatory response model is a classical conditioning model of drug tolerance. This model suggests that environmental stimuli associated with drug intake become linked with the drug's effects on the body to produce a conditioned response opposite to the drug's effect. This is a compensating response designed to maintain bodily homeostasis.

The conditioned appetitive motivational model is a classical conditioning model of craving. According to this model, the conditioned stimuli associated with the positive reinforcing effects of drugs become capable of bringing about a positive motivational state, similar to the one elicited by the drug itself. This state, in turn, creates strong, continuing urges to seek and use the drug and explains why former abusers have such difficulty staying off drugs when they return to the environments where they developed their addictions.

Operant conditioning models have been used to identify differences between alcoholic and nonalcoholic individuals willingness to "work" for alcohol. These differences suggest that in general, alcoholics will work longer and harder to earn alcohol than nonalcoholics. Researchers have applied these finding to the treatment of alcoholism by focusing on providing alternative reinforcement for abstinence.

Vicarious reinforcement and modeling explain the importance of social and peer influences on drinking rates and patterns. Likewise, alcohol expectancies play a major role in predicting alcohol consumption. Alcohol abusers anticipate significantly more pleasure from drinking than nonabusing peers.

Psychopathology and Personality Factors

Psychopathological explanations of substance abuse assume that it occurs, at least partially, because of comorbidity, the presence of two or more psychiatric disorders in a single person. The conditions that often accompany alcohol dependence, for example, are depression and antisocial personality disorder, followed by schizophrenia, anxiety disorders, and sleep disorders. The major problem in this area is the "chicken-and-egg" problem. That is, do the symptoms of the disorder precede the substance abuse, are the consequences of the troubled life of the substance abuser, follow the development of substance abuse, or some combination.

The psychodynamic model of alcoholism and drug dependence portrays these disorders as ultimately unsuccessful efforts to satisfy adulthood dependence needs that were unmet in infancy and early childhood. While this model has not been confirmed with empirical research, the possibility of an addictive personality is considered as important by some researchers. As with the issue of comorbidity, it is difficult to determine if the personality causes the substance abuse or is the result of substance abuse.

A Biopsychosocial Model

This model best fits what we know about substance abuse. Genetic factors play a role in abuse and dependence. Contemporary social learning theory provides an account for why all individuals with this genetic predisposition do not develop substance use problems.

Treatment of Substance Abuse and Dependence

Group and Family Therapy

Group and family therapy have become treatments of choice for substance abuse. Group therapy is popular because it offered therapists a way to confront their patients' denial of the seriousness of their abuse problems. An appealing aspect of family therapy is that it assumes that substance abuse is not the abusers problem alone.

Behavior Therapy

Chemical aversion treatment has consistently shown the most promising of all approaches to treating alcoholism. It is possible that it is so effective because participants must be very motivated in order to participate. Several behavior therapy programs have tested a revolutionary concept, nonabstinent treatment goals. These programs allow participants to learn to control their use of addictive substances rather than to stop totally. Most clinicians today reject the use of controlled drinking goals for chronic alcoholics, due to the lack of supportive research findings. There is more support, though, for the use of nonabstinent drinking goals for drinkers who have just begun to have problems with their drinking. In general it appears that controlled drinking is feasible for early stage problem drinkers, in contrast to chronic alcoholics.

In addition to trying to get individuals to stop drinking, prevention of relapse is also important. Marlatt and Gordon's relapse prevention model addresses this phase of treatment by stressing the importance of identifying the cues in the recovering person's environment that are associated with relapse, and to strengthen coping strategies for dealing with these high risk situations.

Motivational interviewing is also part of the behavioral approach. This technique provides patients direct feedback on present and past drug use to try to help foster willingness of the patient to participate more fully in treatment.

Detoxification

Detoxification is the process of withdrawing a drug-dependent person from substances he or she is addicted to. For high-risk individuals, this process involves a gradual daily-dose reduction, spread over a week or more.

Pharmacological Interventions

Antabuse (disulfiram) blocks the chemical breakdown of alcohol. When even the smallest amount of alcohol is consumed by someone with Antabuse in his or her bloodstream, an acetaldehyde reaction takes place and the individual quickly begins to experience nausea, vomiting, profuse sweating, and markedly increased respiration and heartrate. This is a reaction that most alcoholics say they'd do anything to avoid.

Narcotic antagonist such as naloxone and naltrexone are quite controversial. They bring immediate withdrawal from narcotic drugs. When an addict who is on a maintenance dose of naloxone slips and ingests or injects an opiate like heroin, he will not experience its reinforcing effects.

Methadone is used to treat heroin addiction. It is a synthetic opiate which is used as a replacement for heroin. For most users, methadone produces a less pleasant high.

Many drugs are used to manage withdrawal symptoms including minor tranquilizers such as Librium and Valium. Nicotine gum or tablets and lobeline reduce nicotine-induced withdrawal symptoms. These drugs have had moderately positive results.

Self-Help Groups

Alcoholics anonymous (AA) has been a major factor in alcoholism treatment for some 60 years. Research suggests that this treatment is effective for between 25 and 50% at the 1-year abstinence mark, similar to other treatments. Synanon and Narcotics Anonymous are self-help programs for drug addicts. Narcotics Anonymous is similar to AA while Synanon requires residence in a house during which members confront each other in a constant effort to break down defenses and denial.

Stages of Change in Addictions Treatment

James O. Prochaska concluded that modifying addictive behaviors progresses through five stages of change: precontemplation, contemplation, preparation, action, maintenance. Different specific treatments seem to be most effective at each stage.

Effectiveness of Prevention and Treatment Programs

Efforts over the past 30 years to change public attitudes towards smoking have been very successful; efforts to prevent alcoholism and other drug abuse have been less so. Treatment of alcoholism and drug dependence have been modestly effective. Motivation to change abusive patterns is an especially important determinant of treatment success. Matching patients both to treatments and to therapists has also showed promise.

KEY IDEAS AND OBJECTIVES FOR STUDENTS

After reading the chapter, you should be able to answer each of the following questions:

1. What were historical views of alcoholism and drug abuse?

2. How did the classification of substance disorders differ in DSM-I and DSM-II, DSM-III, DSM-III-R, and DSM-IV

3. What are the prevalence rates for alcohol abuse or dependence? How do they vary with age, sex and ethnicity? How does polysubstance abuse make it difficult to estimate prevalence in the U.S.?

4. What are the consequences of alcohol and drug intoxication in terms of risk for accidents, crime, high-risk sexual behavior, and family violence?

5. What are the physical and health consequences of chronic alcohol and drug abuse?

6. What is the etiology of substance abuse and dependence and which factors are included in etiological explanations? Which perspective provides the best explanation of these problems?

7. What treatments are available for alcohol and drug abuse and dependence?

8. How does the stages of change model affect the success of smoking cessation efforts?

9. How effective are efforts to prevent substance-related disorders? How effective are efforts to reduce the incidence of drunken driving, fetal alcohol syndrome, workplace alcohol problems, and alcohol-related HIV infection?

10. What percentage of alcohol and drug abusers in any given year receive treatment and how many benefit from treatment?

Substance-Related Disorders in the Movies

1. Bright Lights, Big City (1988, MGM/UA, 110 min). This film portrays a self-destructive, cocaine-snorting, would-be writer in New York. The film provides insight into recreational drug use among successful, or semi-successful individuals.

2. Bird (1988, Warner, 163 min) This film is a tribute to the short, tormented life of legendary jazz great Charlie "Bird" Parker. The movie hammers away at the musician's tragic drug abuse that resulted in his untimely death.

3. Boyz N the Hood (1991, Columbia TriStar, 107 min). The story of young African Americans trying to survive a South Central Los Angeles neighborhood. While the focus in on more than drug abuse, this film offers a third perspective to substance abuse in America.

Questions after watching the movies.

1. Given the text's description of substance abuse and substance dependence, for the main character, why would he fit the criteria for substance dependence? which would best be diagnosed as substance abuse?

2. How did the films deal with the cause of the substance use problem? What differences did you observe? What were the major consistencies (or inconsistencies) with contemporary theories?

3. How did the films deal with the issue of "treatment" or "cure"? What were the major consistencies (or inconsistencies) with contemporary theories?

<u>Integrating Perspectives</u>
A Biopsychosocial Model

The Case of Sigmund Freud: Perspectives on Nicotine Dependence

<u>Biological Factors</u>

•Freud was aware of the dangers of cigar smoking and had personal experience with various forms of cancer and precancerous conditions, yet he continued to smoke.

•Attempts to reduce smoking were accompanied with specific physiological changes (heart rate problems). Later in life, his angina was relieved with he stopped smoking. Although he continued to try to sop smoking, he could not.

<u>Psychological Factors</u>

•In general, psychological factors are thought to play a major role in nicotine dependence. Although little information is provided about the Case of Freud, peer pressure and social learning are thought to be quite important.

•For Freud, smoking appeared to relieve the depression that occurred when he stopped smoking.

<u>Social Factors</u>

•Smoking was widely accepted in Freud's culture. It is legal and up until recently, most individuals were quite tolerant of smoking. Today there appears to be more concern with adolescent smoking and exposure to smoke (passive smoking).

Sample Multiple-Choice Questions

1. The first publicly funded treatment programs for alcoholism were called _____.
   a. inebriate asylums
   b. bedlam asylums
   c. laudanum asylums
   d. ethanol asylums

2. Gene has been doing cocaine for 2 years now, spending most of his school loan money buying it whenever he can. Over the last year, Gene has noticed that he needs more and more cocaine to achieve the same high he is used to. In addition, if he doesn't stay high, he experiences restlessness, agitation, and sleeplessness until he gets high again. Gene is suffering from ____________.
   a. substance dependence with physiological dependence
   b. substance dependence without physiological dependence
   c. substance abuse with physiological dependence
   d. substance abuse without physiological dependence

3. Approximately _____ million people in the U.S. meet DSM-IV criteria for alcohol abuse or dependence.
   a. 8-10
   b. 11-13
   c. 14-16
   d. 17-20

4. According to the text, which one of the following statements is NOT an effect of alcohol intoxication?
   a. Heightened risk of having an automobile accident.
   b. Increased risk for home or work-related injuries.
   c. High risk sex behavior.
   d. Permanent, disabling changes in the brain.

5. A committee has been appointed to examine various aspects of drug use, including consumption patterns and trends, health-related costs, deaths associated with use of each drug, etc. The committee has decided to focus their initial efforts on the substance that is attributed to more deaths each year than any other substance. It has also been concluded by experts that this substance produces a dependence greater and more quickly than any of the other substances studied. Which substance will the committee focus its efforts on first?
   a. Alcohol
   b. Crack / cocaine
   c. Nicotine
   d. Heroin

6. Expert ratings of dependence properties in commonly used substances in order of most serious to least serious is _____.
    a. nicotine, heroin, cocaine
    b. alcohol, cocaine, nicotine
    c. cocaine, alcohol, nicotine
    d. cocaine, alcohol, heroin

7. Larry and Harry are twins who have both developed addictions to alcohol, cocaine, and cigarettes. Their father, a wealthy businessman, has demanded that they seek help or else they will be disinherited from the family fortunes. Larry and Harry join a substance abuse treatment program. They meet weekly with their therapist and a few other people with similar substance dependencies. In these weekly meetings, Larry and Harry are confronted about their drug problems. In particular, they are forced to confront their denial of the problems and the seriousness of them. This type of therapy is called _____.
    a. family therapy
    b. group therapy
    c. motivational therapy
    d. relapse prevention therapy

8. Rick is in a smoking cessation program. Over the past few weeks, Rick has cut back on the number of cigarettes he smokes each day. Rick is probably in the _____ stage of change.
    a. precontemplation
    b. contemplation
    c. preparation
    d. action

9. Fetal alcohol syndrome is linked to alcohol consumption of ______________.
    a. the mother
    b. the father
    c. both parents
    d. the child

10. No more than _______ percent of alcohol dependent individuals enter treatment in any given year.
    a. 10
    b. 15
    c. 20
    d. 25

Answer Key

1. a
2. a
3. c
4. d
5. c
6. a
7. b
8. c
9. a
10. a

CHAPTER 10 PSYCHOLOGICAL FACTORS AFFECTING HEALTH

This chapter reviews the area of behavioral medicine and health psychology. An historical perspective is presented, followed by three models to explain the link between stress and illness. Psychological effects on immune system and cardiovascular functioning are examined, and factors associated with health are presented in the context of obesity and AIDS. Finally, prevention and treatment are addressed. The chapter opens with the case of Barbara Boggs Sigmund, who died of cancer; this case is used to raise issues relevant to linking psychological and physical factors.

A Historical Overview

Physical disorders affected by psychological factors were previously considered psychosomatic disorders which resulted from unconscious emotional conflicts. Conflicts involving passivity and dependence versus independence and achievement were thought to lead to ulcers and colitis. Repressed hostility was thought to be related to hypertension, migraine headaches and coronary heart disease. This view was not based on empirical investigation, however, and had little influence.

Behavioral medicine is the integration of behavioral and biomedical sciences in order to understand, prevent, and treat physical illness. This field emerged in the 1970s from the behavior therapy and its application to physical problems. It is concerned with specific interventions and tends to be interdisciplinary, involving both behavioral scientists and medical professionals. Health psychology overlaps with behavioral medicine in that it addresses interventions; however, it also encompasses socioenvironmental factors and individual differences affecting health and illness, as well as health policy and the health care system. Health psychology is based solely on the discipline of psychology. These two branches are consistent with a biopsychosocial model, which emphasizes the interactive influences of multiple factors.

The Relationship Between Mental Health & Physical Health

It is difficult to determine the direction of the relationship between psychological and physical factors. A longitudinal study by Vaillant (1979) found that mental health has a direct influence on physical health, even when factors such as cigarette smoking, obesity, and parents' longevity are controlled. Poor mental health predicts premature aging and deterioration in physical health.

Stress and Illness

Individuals exposed to severe psychological stress are less healthy and develop more physical illnesses than those with less stress. Risk factors are characteristics that increase the likelihood that an individual will get an illness, even though the reason for the increased risk may be unclear. Stress can be defined in terms of complex physiological responses, or as specific stimuli or environmental conditions which influence persons in similar ways. Hans

Selye proposed a response model in which he conceptualized stress as a nonspecific body response that follows three stages.
These stages are: 1) alarm and mobilization reaction involving arousal of the autonomic nervous system; 2) resistance involving the body's attempts to adapt to the physiological demands placed on it; and 3) exhaustion involving death or irreversible damage due to prolonged exposure to the harmful stimulation. This sequence of physiological responses has been found to occur in response to both psychological and physical stress.

Both the hypothalamus and the limbic system control emotions and motivation. The hypothalamus influences both the autonomic nervous system and the endocrine system. The autonomic nervous system is mobilized in response to emotion or stress. The hypothalamus secretes hormones to stimulate the pituitary gland, which then acts in concert with the hypothalamus to control emotional responses, hunger, thirst, digestion, and sexual behavior. The pituitary gland also activates the adrenal gland (which is also stimulated by the autonomic nervous system); corticosteroids and catecholamines are secreted by the adrenal gland in response to stress, and these hormones influence brain functioning. The limbic system includes the hippocampus, which plays a major role in memory. The hippocampus is particularly responsive to corticosteroids released by the adrenal cortex and helps turn off the stress response. Figure 10.1 on p. 327 is a diagram of the stress response.

Stimulus models of stress identify particular events or conditions which are assumed to affect persons adversely. Cohen proposed four categories of stressors: acute stressors; stressor sequences triggered by particular events; chronic stressors; and chronic but intermittent stressors. Holmes & Rahe have attempted to identify stressful life events, both positive and negative, which are assumed to produce varying degrees of stress (see Table 10.2 on p. 328). This approach is problematic because not all stressors are included (e.g., some chronic stressors, daily hassles), because the direction of the link between the stressor and illness cannot be determined, and because individuals react very differently to the same stressor.

A biopsychosocial model is needed to identify multiple factors which account for differences in response to positive versus negative events, and for individual differences in responsivity to the same stimulus. Cognitive appraisal of a stressful event can affect the impact of the stressor. Lazarus proposed that a stressor is evaluated for potential threat according to harm already incurred, threat of future harm, and challenge involving potential for personal gain from future events. A person's explanatory style, or typical manner of explaining the negative life events they experience, is also related to physical illness. Attributing the causes of negative events to stable, global and internal factors characterizes a pessimistic style which is associated with poor health. Both cognitive and behavioral coping can mediate the effects of stress. Active, or problem-focused coping involves attempts to change a stressful situation directly; this may be effective when the person actually has some control over aspects of the stressful situation. Passive, or emotion-focused coping involves acceptance and management of feelings; this is most helpful in situations over which one has little or no control.

Social support also mediates the relationship between stress and illness. Epidemiological studies have consistently found a link between social support and mortality rate. Social support may act as a protective factor or buffer against negative biological effects of stress. Alternatively, social support may directly enhance health by fostering a sense of meaning of life, and/or it may indirectly enhance health by encouraging health-promoting behaviors (e.g., getting enough sleep, following a beneficial diet, avoiding drug use, etc.). However, the perceived quality of social support is strongly influenced by genetic factors which may affect the selection of particular social environments.

Psychological Effects on Biological Mechanisms

There are two major ways in which psychological factors affect health. First, these factors affect the basic biological mechanisms and functions that mediate illness and disease. Second, they determine specific health-promoting and health-damaging behaviors, such as quitting cigarette smoking and adopting safe-sex practices. Diseases related to the immune system and metabolic diseases provide a good model for the effects of psychological factors on health.

The immune system protects against viral and bacterial disease through two basic components. Humoral immunity involves the release of antibodies into the blood and body fluids to defend against bacteria and viruses; B-cells and plasma cells are involved in this process. Cellular immunity protects against viruses, cancer cells, and foreign tissues by releasing T-cells. Natural killer (NK) cells destroy viruses and some tumor cells; imbalance in this system may result in autoimmune diseases.

Stress reduces both humoral and cellular immune responses. Lack of control over the stressor may be especially harmful to the immune responses. Decreases in T-cell and NK cell activity have been observed following examinations, bereavement, and divorce. Perceived control over the stressors may protect one against immunosuppressive effects of stress. Stress can increase susceptibility to viral infections like colds, and the greater the stress the greater the likelihood of developing a cold when exposed to a cold virus. Psychological factors may also affect some forms of cancer in some patients. Women with breast cancer who participated in a psychotherapy group and used self-hypnosis to control pain lived almost twice as long as those in a control group. The likelihood of developing colorectal cancer has been linked to the degree of work-related stress. Stress may affect cancer by impairing the immune system through lesions in DNA. These findings, however, should not be interpreted as evidence that psychological factors alone account for the development and/or cure of cancer or other diseases.

Acquired immune deficiency syndrome (AIDS) occurs when the human immunodeficiency virus (HIV) infects a person and the cells of the immune system are attacked. The fact that some people who acquire HIV or AIDS live for 5 or more years suggests that psychosocial factors may influence the onset and course of the disease through effects on the immune system. This may occur by reducing the negative effects of stress on immune function. Increased autonomic arousal is linked to release of catecholamines which enhance NK activity. However, stressful life events and depression have not been found to affect immune functioning in AIDS patients.

Cardiovascular disease includes hypertension (chronic high blood pressure) and heart disease. Hypertension can cause stroke, heart disease, and kidney damage and is caused by genetic, dietary, and sociocultural factors. Thus, the biopsychosocial perspective is very useful in understanding the disease. Genetic factors predispose persons to respond to stress with greater increases in blood pressure; blacks tend to show greater autonomic reactivity than whites, which could explain the greater prevalence among blacks. Psychological factors include anxiety, which increases the risk for developing hypertension. High sodium intake and excessive alcohol consumption are also risk factors for hypertension. Sociocultural factors such as industrialization are associated with increased risk for hypertension, and exposure to greater levels of unemployment, poverty, and crime could also explain the high prevalence among blacks.

Coronary heart disease (CHD) is characterized by an inherited biological tendency which interacts with physiological, nutritional, and environmental factors. Psychological factors such as a hostile or aggressive response to stress, feeling under time pressures, competitive and ambitious styles, otherwise known as Type A personality characteristics, have been linked to CHD. While early studies suggested that Type A behavioral styles increased risk for CHD, more recent studies have shown that hostility appears to be the important component, while other components of Type A behavior do not increase risk for CHD. Stress can lead to CHD by accelerating the buildup of plaque in arteries. In cases of acute stressful events, a rupture of the atherosclerotic plaque can cause a blood clot which can block bloodflow and cause sudden death. Depression can also increase the negative effects of cigarette smoking and higher than normal levels of fibrinogen (which facilitates plaque formation in arteries), thereby increasing the risk for CHD.

Diabetes is a metabolic disorder in which the metabolism of carbohydrates and regulation of blood-sugar levels is impaired. This can lead to increased risk of heart disease and stroke, blindness, susceptibility to infection, and loss of sexual functioning. Type I, or insulin-dependent, diabetes occurs when the body lacks sufficient insulin because insulin-producing cells in the pancreas degenerate. Type II diabetes occurs mainly among obese adults and is characterized by sufficient levels of insulin, but the insulin is metabolically ineffective in converting glucose into energy. Type II diabetes occurs most often in obese people who have a positive family history of the disease. Stress directly affects diabetes by influencing how well people adhere to a behavioral treatment program. Stress also affects diabetes indirectly. First, cortisol and catecholamines are released into the bloodstream in response to perceived stress, which leads the pancreas to release glycogen, which is converted into glucose by the liver. Second, cortisol and catecholamines block the release of insulin from the pancreas, which increases levels of circulating glucose.

Psychological Determinants of Health-Promoting and Health-Damaging Behaviors

Adherence to health-promoting behaviors, such as exercising, reducing fat intake, avoiding smoking, avoiding unprotected sex, is poor. Only about half of all patients follow their doctors' advice regarding referral advice; many drop out of care, take insufficient medication or take medication on an irregular basis. Adherence to medical intervention may enhance health in other ways. Simply taking medication faithfully, even when the medication was a placebo, was linked to improved health and survival, even when disease severity was controlled. It has been proposed that the act of adhering activates self-efficacy and related coping responses that also lead to improved health outcomes.

Obesity is increasingly common, with 1 in 3 adults in the U.S. overweight. Obesity is defined as being 20% or more above one's desirable weight. Obesity occurs most frequently among black non-Hispanic women and Mexican-American women. Consequences of obesity include hypertension, diabetes, pulmonary and kidney problems, osteoarthritis, some types of cancer and complications in recovery from surgery. It is also an independent risk factor for cardiovascular disease in men and women. Abdominal obesity (fat storage greater above the waist) is associated with the greatest increased risk for disease and death, while femoral obesity (fat storage greater below the waist) is associated with less risk. Twin and adoption studies have supported a genetic predisposition toward obesity. The set-point theory of body weight assumes that individuals have a biologically programmed weight range and one's body acts to defend particular weight ranges. Genetically determined metabolic rate may be one mechanism which affects body weight, with low metabolic rate increasing one's risk for obesity. Once obesity occurs, it is maintained by irreversible formation of fat cells and an increase in metabolic efficiency. Obesity is about six times more common among women of low SES than high SES. In fact, the SES level into which a woman is born is almost as strong a correlate of obesity as her own SES level. Since blacks have lower SES than whites, on average, this might partially explain the greater rate of obesity among blacks.

The most effective treatments include several components: behavior modification to alter eating habits, nutritional counseling to increase knowledge about diet and health, self-control strategies to achieve lifestyle change, cognitive restructuring to change unhealthy attitudes about body weight and shape, and increased physical exercise to promote fitness. These treatments result in an average weight loss of 30-40 pounds over a 6-month period. Although effective in the short term, treatments are relatively ineffective in the long term. About 2/3 of obese adult patients who lost weight maintained their weight loss at 1-year follow-up; however, 90-95% had returned to baseline weight within 5 years. Relapse usually occurs when patients abandon the nutrition and behavioral strategies learned in treatment. Children who are obese, however, are more likely to maintain weight loss. This may occur because it is easier to change eating and activity habits in children than in adults, and/or because parents can exert external control over their children through social support and food management, whereas adults do not have that external control.

AIDS is now the second leading cause of death among U.S. males aged 18-44 years. The prevalence of HIV among gay men and intravenous drug abusers is high. However, heterosexuals and women are contracting the disease at increasing rates. Initially, significant behavioral changes in the gay male population occurred in response to community-based activism which promoted education, social norms and support for safe-sex practices, and modeling and social reinforcement facilitated these changes. IV drug users have been less successful in reducing the rate at which they share needles or stop drug use. They typically lack the means for behavior change, including effective treatment of drug use, access to sterile needles, educational and financial resources. They are also frequently involved in illegal activities and have little social support. Even those who use safer injections do not change their sex practices. Condoms may not be used because they are often associated with the breakup of heterosexual relationships, perhaps because they signal that one partner has HIV and/or raise concerns with sexual fidelity. The majority of IV drug users are male, who infect female partners, who may transmit the infection to infants during pregnancy. Minority groups living in poor communities with high drug use are at particular risk for AIDS.

Prevention and Treatment of Health-Damaging Behaviors

Psychosomatic medicine in the 1940s and 1950s applied psychodynamic therapy to resolve unconscious conflicts which affect medical conditions. Psychodynamic treatment is still used today, as well as cognitive-behavioral treatments; biofeedback and relaxation training are among the most common.

Biofeedback developed after it was discovered that physiological functions regulated by the autonomic nervous system (heartrate and blood pressure) could be classically conditioned and modified through operant conditioning. Biofeedback is the direct modification of physiological responses (e.g., blood pressure) by feedback that makes the person aware of the process. Tension headaches (painful contractions of skeletal muscles of the face, scalp, neck, and shoulders in response to psychological stress) are effectively reduced by EMG feedback, although the exact mechanism of change is still unclear.

Progressive muscle relaxation is widely used to treat stress-related disorders by alternate tensing and relaxing of different muscle groups. Jacobson's method, which is exclusively somatic, teaches a person to become aware of feelings of tension and to replace them by relaxation; this method can take months or years to master. A brief method emphasizes a suggestion of relaxation (a cognitive component) and takes only 4 to 10 sessions. Both methods represent a coping skill in which a person can identify early signs of stress and then respond with relaxation skills. Transcendental meditation is a form of training in which the person adopts a passive attitude and focuses on a single object (e.g., a mantra or chant). Relaxation training has been used successfully to treat asthma, tension headaches, migraines, hypertension, Type A behavior pattern, chronic pain, and insomnia. It has also been used to reduce stress of those with cancer to control the nausea and vomiting experienced prior to chemotherapy.

Interventions for multiple risk factors are aimed at entire communities, rather than individuals. The Stanford Three-Community Study was a two-year, broad intervention program to reduce risk of coronary heart disease in two communities. One community received a media-based intervention. A second community received the media-based intervention supplemented by an intensive program of face-to-face instruction in behavior change for participants at high risk for CHD. The third served as a control. Social-cognitive theory and behavioral self-control principles of self-monitoring, modeling, and reinforcement were the content of the programs. Results showed that subjects in both intervention communities gained knowledge about risk factors for CHD and the media-based program in the first community produced changes in self-reported levels of cholesterol and fats. The intensive instruction plus media program in the second community achieved the best results: risk for CHD was lowered significantly, primarily through reduced cigarette smoking. Compared to the control community, treated communities showed significant reductions in systolic blood pressure and dietary cholesterol; the second also had significantly lowered plasma cholesterol. The Stanford Five-City Project extended the findings of the Three Community study. The study lasted 5 to 6 years, included more diverse populations and focused more intensively on grass-root community organization to promote healthy behavior. Monterey and Salinas received continual education about cardiovascular risk factors (reducing cholesterol level, blood pressure, body weight, and cigarette smoking, and increasing physical activity). Modesto, San Luis Obispo, and Santa Maria received no intervention. Results confirmed that risk factors for heart disease could be altered. Monterey and Salinas communities showed greater reductions in plasma cholesterol, blood pressure, and rate of cigarette smoking compared to the three control cities. Overall risk of heart disease was reduced by 16 percent in the two cities, but there were minimal effects on weight loss. More recently, Haskell and associates demonstrated the efficacy of intervention for multiple risk factors with a group of 300 men and women with coronary artery disease. Intervention subjects reduced fat intake, lost weight, increased physical exercise, reduced cigarette smoking, and reduced cholesterol through diet and medication. Patients receiving routine medical care showed no changes in risk factors.

KEY IDEAS AND OBJECTIVES FOR STUDENTS

After reading the chapter, you should be able to answer each of the following questions:

1. What was the view of psychosomatic medicine during the 1940s and 1950s?

2. What was the emphasis of the fields of behavioral medicine and health psychology and how did they differ from the psychoanalytic approach?

3. What is today's biopsychosocial perspective of health and illness?

4. How do serious emotional problems, such as anxiety or depression, affect risk of developing diseases and dying?

5. How do individuals who are exposed to severe stress in their lives differ from who are not severely stressed?

6. What are the three stages of response to stress, according to the response model?

7. What is the definition of stress according to the stimulus model? What are the four kinds of stressors?

8. What is the biopsychosocial model of stress? How are individual differences in response to stressors explained?,

9. How do psychological factors influence physical health?

10. What are the direct effects on health and illness of psychological factors? How does this influence work?

11. What is the link between stress and cardiovascular diseases such as hypertension and coronary hearth disease (CHD)? How can differences in rates of hypertension between blacks and whites be explained?

12. What is the Type A behavior pattern and how is it linked to CHD?

13. How does stress contribute to heart problems and what are the mechanisms involved?

14. How do psychological factors influence metabolic diseases, such as diabetes, both directly and indirectly?

15. What is adherence and how does it affect health-promoting behaviors?

16. How is obesity defined? Is there a genetic predisposition? How difficult is it to product lasting change in obesity?

17. What is AIDS and what efforts have been made to halt its spread? Have these efforts been successful with all populations?

18. What methods are used by clinicians to prevent and treat health-damaging behaviors?

Psychological Factors Affecting Health in the Movies

1. Falling Down (1993, Warner, 113 min) The opening scene of this movie is an excellent demonstration of autonomic arousal in response to environmental stressors. The character portrayed by Michael Douglas is caught in a traffic jam on a hot summer day. The signs of autonomic arousal include dilating pupils, increased respiration, perspiration, and apparent subjective stress. This segment could help students to apply the biological mechanisms of stress (e.g., Fig. 10.1 on p. 327 in the text). Alternatively, students could identify how they concluded that the character finds the situation stressful. This could then be tied to cognitive factors and the biopsychosocial model of stress.

2. Philadelphia Story (1993, Columbia TriStar, 125 min) This movie portrays the challenges faced by a man with AIDS. When it is discovered by his employers that he has AIDS, he is fired from a successful law firm. His subsequent fight to regain his job and the negative effects of AIDS (including his death) are shown in the context of societal attitudes and stigma associated with this disease. This movie can serve as an illustration of AIDS and could prompt consideration of the issues regarding blaming the victims of physical illnesses that are "preventable." This fits with the case of Barbara Boggs Sigmund presented in the text.

Sample Multiple-Choice Questions

1. Before publication in the DSM third and fourth editions, "physical factors influencing medical conditions" were known as ______________ disorders.
   a. psychosomatic
   b. myocardial
   c. biopsychosocial
   d. pathological

2. The biopsychosocial perspective on health and illness _________.
   a. emphasizes biology and disease
   b. emphasizes the interactive effects of biology and disease
   c. is broader in focus and emphasizes interactive effects
   d. has been replaced by the biomedical model

3. A(n) _________ is a characteristic that increases the likelihood that an individual will get an illness, even though the reason for this increase may be unclear.
   a. adherence factor
   b. risk factor
   c. disease factor
   d. co-morbid factor

4. Hans Selye conceptualized stress as a provoked, nonspecific body response following predictable stages. The three stages are ________.
   a. excitement, hesitation, exhaustion
   b. alarm, reaction, extinguished behavior
   c. frustration, pressure, exhaustion
   d. alarm, resistance, exhaustion

5. The stress proposed by Cohen et al. in which stressors as classified as acute, stressor sequences, chronic stressors, or as chronic but intermittent stressors, is a ___________ model.
   a. response
   b. stimulus
   c. social
   d. cognitive

6. Holly does not have a very smooth relationship with her family. Every Sunday, her family meets in order to go to church together. Like clockwork, at least two of the family members fight with each other each time they meet. Which type of stressor is Holly exposed to?
   a. acute stressor
   b. stressor triggered by a particular event
   c. chronic stressor
   d. chronic but intermittent stressor

7. A person with a pessimistic explanatory style believes that events are caused by ____________ factors.
   a. internal, global, and stable
   b. external, specific, and unstable
   c. harm, threat, and challenge
   d. danger, security, and support

8. Charles has a suppressed immune system due to a great deal of job stress. What two components of the system will have decreased functioning?
   a. humoral and cellular
   b. cellular and molecular
   c. cellular and organ
   d. organ and system

9. Cathy has chronic, abnormally high blood pressure. This is called ________.
   a. autonomic reactivity
   b. hypertension
   c. hypotension
   d. atherosclerosis

10. Studies have shown that approximately _____ percent of patients follow their doctors' advice.
   a. 25
   b. 40
   c. 50
   d. 75

Answer Key

1. a
2. c
3. b
4. d
5. b
6. d
7. a
8. a
9. b
10. c

CHAPTER 11 EATING DISORDERS

Description

Eating disorders are characterized by severe disturbances in eating behavior, maladaptive and unhealthy efforts to control body weight, and abnormal attitudes about body weight and shape. The two most thoroughly studied eating disorders are anorexia nervosa and bulimia nervosa. Other eating disorders that are closely related but do not meet all the diagnostic criteria are classified as eating disorders not otherwise specified (EDNOS). The most common example of EDNOS is binge-eating disorder where there is recurrent binge eating but without the inappropriate weight-control behaviors. Figure 11.1 on page 356 shows the relationship among the types of eating disorders. Note: obesity is not considered a psychiatric disorder. The body mass index (BMI) value is used to determine healthy and unhealthy body weights (weight in kilograms divided by height in meters).

Types of Eating Disorders

Anorexia Nervosa is an eating disorder characterized by a serious loss of weight and disturbed body image. It is divided into two subtypes based on the nature of binge eating and purging. Binge eating has two defining features: 1) consumption of unusually large amounts of food in excess of what most people would eat during similar periods of time and under similar circumstances and, 2) a sense of loss of control over eating. Purging refers to self-induced vomiting or laxative misuse designed to influence body weight and shape. Binge-eating/purging type involves regular episodes of binge eating and purging; these individuals alternate between periods of rigid control and impulsive behavior, display significantly more psychopathology, and are more likely to attempt suicide. If binge eating and purging do not occur regularly, this is referred to as restricting type. These individuals are highly controlled, rigid, and often obsessive. The box on page 357 lists the DSM-IV Diagnostic Criteria for Anorexia Nervosa.

Associated Psychopathology. The most common form of psychopathology associated with anorexia nervosa is depression. Rates of co-occurrence range from 21 to 91 percent. Also co-occurs with anxiety disorders, in particular obsessive-compulsive disorder where obsessional tendencies have been reported to predate the development of anorexia nervosa and to exist after weight restoration. Substance abuse is also common in patients with anorexia nervosa; rates of co-occurrence range form 6.7 to 23 percent; higher levels of substance abuse occur among individuals with the binge-eating/purging subtype. Personality disorders are also associated with anorexia nervosa; rates range from 27 to 93 percent; most strongly associated with cluster C personality (avoidant, dependent, and obsessive-compulsive).

Medical Complications. Medical complications can emerge as a result of starvation and malnutrition. Common physical signs include dry, sometimes yellowish skin, lanugo (fine, downy hair) on the trunk, face, and extremities, sensitivity to cold, cardiovascular problems such as hypotension (low blood pressure), and bradycardia (slow heart beat). Self-induced vomiting may cause the salivary glands to become enlarged, dental enamel to erode, chronic dehydration and electrolyte imbalance. In particular, depletion of serum potassium may lead to hypokalemia, increasing the risk of both renal (kidney) failure and cardiac arrhythmia (irregular heartbeat). As many as 10 percent die from medical complications or suicide.

Bulimia Nervosa is an eating disorder characterized by binge eating, extreme methods of weight control, and abnormal attitudes about the importance of body weight and shape. In contrast to previous diagnostic systems, the DSM-IV identifies two subtypes of bulimia: purging and nonpurging. Evidence suggests that the purging type is a more severe and chronic form. Individuals with bulimia show a cognitive style marked by rigid rules and all-or-nothing thinking--either completely in control or out of control, virtuous or indulgent. Bulimia nervosa usually begins in adolescence or early adulthood. Binge eating develops during or after a period of restrictive dieting, which is followed closely by purging. Lifetime prevalence ranges from 1 to 2 percent among adolescent and young adult women. Bulimia nervosa can be effectively treated in the majority of cases, with good prospects for a full and lasting recovery. The box on page 360 lists the DSM-IV Diagnostic Criteria for Bulimia Nervosa.

Associated Psychopathology. Bulimia nervosa is strongly associated with other disorders in clinical samples. Co-occurrence with depression is so frequent that it is hypothesized that the two disorders share a common etiology. However, depression usually disappears following successful treatment of the eating disorder; therefore, depression is perhaps a consequence, not a cause. Anxiety disorders also co-occur frequently with bulimia nervosa, especially generalized anxiety disorder and social phobia. Substance abuse is also associated with bulimia nervosa; lifetime prevalence of substance abuse in patients with bulimia nervosa ranges from 9 to 55 percent. This co-occurrence was found in the general population and among individuals with substance abuse problems.

Medical Complications. As with anorexia nervosa, it is the purging that can produce negative health effects. Physical complaints such as fatigue, headaches, and puffy cheeks (due to enlargement of salivary glands as a result of repeated vomiting). The most serious medical complications are probably posed by electrolyte abnormalities (low potassium) which can disrupt heart rate and cause kidney failure. Use of ipecac to induce vomiting and excessive laxative abuse can lead to dependence on these medications and cause severe constipation or even permanent damage to the colon. It is important to medically screen individuals who purge and have blood tests to assess electrolyte status and fluid imbalances.

Binge-Eating Disorder is an eating disorder characterized by recurrent binge eating but not inappropriate weight-control behaviors. Preliminary data indicate that BED occurs predominantly in individuals who are obese (referred to as "compulsive overeaters" in the clinical and popular literature). Obese patients with BED consume significantly more food than obese nonbingers. BED patients also report disorganized and chaotic eating habits. Controversy over the inclusion of BED in the DSM continues; inclusion was based on two studies which used self-report questionnaires which may have yielded unreliable estimates of binge eating. Binge-eating Disorder is not an official disorder in DSM-IV, but proposed criteria are listed in the DSM-IV table on page 365.

Associated Psychopathology. Obese individuals who binge show significantly greater levels of psychopathology than obese nonbingers (e.g., 60% lifetime prevalence of affective disorders and 70% lifetime rate of anxiety disorders in sample of obese binge eaters). BED does not seem to be significantly associated with alcohol abuse.

Causes

Genetic factors. Family and twin studies show a familial transmission where these disorders are more common among biological relatives of patients with eating disorders than among the general population. The concordance rate for anorexia nervosa in identical twins was 55% and the rate in fraternal twins was only 7% Genetic predisposition may be expressed through certain types of personality structures. In patients with anorexia nervosa, personality traits seem to cluster: obsessional tendencies, rigidity, emotional restraint, preference for familiarity, and poor adaptability to change.

Biological factors. Changes in eating behavior can have significant effects on how the nervous system works; it is difficult to determine whether the biological abnormalities seen in patients with eating disorders result from or cause disturbed eating habits. Serotonin plays a key role in regulating mood and eating behaviors. The available evidence is mixed regarding lower levels of serotonin in those who binge eat. Familial history of psychopathology also plays a role. A family history of depression or substance abuse is a risk factor for bulimia nervosa. Personal and family history of being overweight are both specific risk factors for bulimia nervosa; 10% of individuals with bulimia nervosa have this history, and these factors have been found to be the only two predictors of outcome. Attributable risk is the proportion of cases in the population that are due to the risk factor. The greater the severity of the obesity, the stronger the risk factor.

Dieting. Dieting is closely linked to the onset and maintenance of eating disorders. Various biological, cognitive, and affective consequences may predispose persons to binge eating. A biological factor may be short-term dieting that can reduce serotonin functioning in the brain. Cognitive factors include: unrealistic, rigid standards; vulnerability to loss of control if a diet is broken, which can lead to all-or-nothing reactions. The abstinence violation effect is when individuals attribute their lapses to a complete inability to maintain control and, thus, abandon all attempts to regulate food intake and overeat. Dieting is a risk factor but is not a necessary causal condition for the development of an eating disorder. In contrast to individuals with bulimia nervosa, binge eating often precedes dieting in individuals with BED.

Psychological Factors. Using a case-control design in which a person with an identified clinical disorder is matched with a control subject of the same sex, age, and socioeconomic status, researchers at Oxford University in England were able to collect data about eating disorders from community-based samples. This remedied the problem of representativeness of previous research on the influence of personal and familial factors in the etiology of eating disorders in which only clinical samples where studied. Empirical support for childhood sexual abuse as a general risk factor for psychopathology, but not a specific risk factor for bulimia nervosa, was found. Specific risk factors for eating disorders included negative self-evaluation, perfectionism, and shyness with attributable risks of 11%, 13%, and 15%, respectively.

Stress of Adolescence. Both anorexia nervosa and bulimia nervosa typically develop among girls during adolescence. Adolescence seems to be a period during which females have lower self-esteem, are more concerned with their appearance, and are more vulnerable to affective disturbances than males. Postpubertal changes in body weight and shape are more stressful for females than males, and self-images of female adolescents are more interpersonally oriented.

The Role of the Family. Minuchin and colleagues (1978) identified a characteristic pattern of interaction in families of adolescents with anorexia nervosa: enmeshment (members overinvolved with one another, personal boundaries are crossed), overprotectiveness, rigidity, and conflict avoidance and poor conflict resolution. Daughters with anorexia nervosa are either the object of diverted conflict for parents or are drawn into coalition with one parent against the other. Criticism, contradictory communication, and family focus on the importance of body shape and weight in eating disorder families represent specific risk factors. Other specific risk factors include frequent parental absence, underinvolvement, high expectations, criticism, and discord between parents.

Social/Cultural Factors. The current cultural context defines the ideal female body shape as thin and lithe. This trend started with the model Twiggy at the end of the 1960s. Evidence of the increasing preference for thinness may be observed in the declining average weights of Playboy centerfolds and Miss America contestants from the late 1950s to late 1970s. The average weight of women in the general population has actually increased by 5 pounds over the same 20-year period. This clash between biological reality and psychosocial pressure is the key to understanding eating disorders. The majority of young women in the U.S. are dissatisfied with their body shapes and weights; most consider themselves overweight even though they are at normal or below-normal weights ("normative discontent"). Over 60% of adolescent females diet. Being thin is particularly important among white, middle- and upper-class women. Obesity is strongly and inversely correlated with socioeconomic status for women, but not for men. There is a positive correlation between cultural pressure to be thin and prevalence of eating disorders. Eating disorders are most common among white, upper-socioeconomic-level females and among individuals in specific occupations and activities that place pressure on females to be thin.

Treatment

Anorexia Nervosa. The medical complications brought about by reaching dangerously low weights often require hospitalization. The first goal is to restore individuals to near normal body weight. This can usually be achieved with therapeutic support and carefully planned nutritional treatment. More drastic interventions, such as tube feeding, are only necessary in the most resistant patients whose lives are at risk. Behavior modification has proven effective in increasing the rate of weight gain during hospitalization; treatment consists of providing positive reinforcements for gradual weight gain (e.g., visiting privileges, activities). Patients tend to relapse and lose weight, however, necessitating readmission to the hospital. Family therapy is one of the most commonly employed approaches. It is based on the assumption that the functioning of a patient's family is disturbed and serves to maintain her eating disorder, so the entire family is involved in the therapy. This treatment lacks empirical support. Individual psychotherapy typically consists of some form of psychodynamic treatment. Crisp and colleagues (1994) have the most promising approach to date. It is based on the assumption that anorexia nervosa is a phobia about normal weight gain caused by conflict over becoming a mature woman; the eating disorder is a maladaptive way of coping with this emotional conflict. Therapy is aimed at helping patients develop more constructive ways of coping with their psychosexual development. Drug therapy has included neuroleptic (antipsychotic) and antidepressant drugs. This has produced only marginal effects in promoting weight gain.

Bulimia Nervosa

Medication. Antidepressant drugs, such as imipramine and desipramine (tricyclics) and fluoxetine (Prozac) have proven effective. These drugs treat the depression that is commonly associated with bulimia nervosa. Problems with using these drugs include the following: many individuals are reluctant to take medication; more persons drop out of pharmacotherapy because of the side effects caused by the drugs; individuals tend to relapse quickly when the drugs are withdrawn.

Psychological Treatment. Cognitive-behavioral therapy (CBT) is the most intensively studied and is superior to antidepressant medication. It typically consists of 16 to 20 sessions administered over a 4- to 5-month period. CBT is aimed at normalizing the chaotic eating patterns, modifying abnormal attitudes about shape and weight, and equipping persons with more constructive coping skills for handling stressful life events. CBT produces an average reduction in binge eating and purging that ranges form 73 to 93%. Roughly 50% of treated patients stop these behaviors. CBT also reduces unhealthy dietary restraints and helps patients become more accepting of their body shapes and weights. Improvements have been maintained for up to 1 year. Interpersonal psychotherapy (IPT) is a time-limited treatment approach that focuses on the individual's current social functioning, interpersonal conflicts, and role transitions. It is not as effective as CBT immediately following treatment, but is equally effective at 1- and 6-year follow-ups.

Binge-Eating Disorder. Preliminary studies have shown both antidepressant medication and psychological treatment to significantly reduce binge eating in patients with BED. The two most promising psychological approaches are CBT and IPT. These treatments appear to reduce binge eating but do not promote weight loss.

KEY IDEAS AND OBJECTIVES FOR STUDENTS

After reading the chapter, you should be able to answer each of the following questions:

1. What are the characteristics and symptoms of anorexia nervosa?

2. What are the characteristics and symptoms of bulimia nervosa?

3. What are the characteristics and symptoms of binge-eating disorder (BED)?

4. Do anorexia and bulimia nervosa run in families, and how is this influenced?

5. Do the biological abnormalities seen in patients with eating disorders result from or cause the disturbed behavior?

6. How is dieting related to the development of eating disorders?

7. What are the risk factors for bulimia nervosa?

8. How do current cultural norms about the ideal female body affect dieting and risk for eating disorders? What gender differences exist?

9. What is the first goal of treatment for patients with anorexia nervosa? What types of therapy are often used? How successful is each therapy?

10. Which treatments are effective in treating bulimia nervosa and BED? Which treatments result in broad and lasting improvement?

Using Case Studies in Abnormal Psychology by Meyer & Osborne
The Eating Disorders

General Summary

Chapter 11 in the casebook presents case material on anorexia nervosa and bulimia nervosa. Characteristics of each disorder are reviewed, as well as suggestions for appropriate diet, food intake and eating habits. The case of Karen Carpenter is used to illustrate anorexia nervosa which is resistant to treatment and which eventually led to her death. The case of Princess Diana is used to illustrate the course of bulimia nervosa and associated characteristics. Both cases examine precipitating factors (e.g., family characteristics) and treatments.

Case Comparisons

Anorexia Nervosa: The Case of Karen Carpenter. The development and relatively late onset of anorexia nervosa is examined in the context of family characteristics, Karen's individual personality characteristics, and life stresses. The diagnostic criteria for anorexia nervosa are summarized on page 357 of the text. Provide a summary of the specific characteristics of Karen that support this diagnosis. Are any of the criteria questionable? What factors (family characteristics, personality characteristics of Karen, stress) appeared to contribute to the development of this disorder. Which theoretical models are linked to these factors? What treatment options were used by Karen? Were any of these effective? What treatment, if any, could have prevented her death?

Bulimia Nervosa: The Case of Princess Diana. The development of bulimia nervosa and other associated difficulties (e.g., suicidal behaviors, self-injury) is examined in this case. The diagnostic criteria for bulimia nervosa are presented on page 360 of the text. Provide a summary of the specific characteristics of Princess Diana that support the diagnosis using each of the criteria. Are any of the criteria questionable? Did Princess Diana exhibit symptoms of any other disorders (e.g., major depression)? Support your answer with specific symptoms. What factors may have led to the development of this problem for Diana? Which theoretical models are linked to these factors? Which treatment options were used by Princess Diana? Which of the multiple treatments do you believe to be responsible for her improvement and why?

Integrating Perspectives
A Biopsychosocial Model

The Case of Karen Carpenter

Biological Factors

•"Large hips" were thought to run in her family. Karen's mother felt that there was "no getting rid of them."
•Karen weighed 145 pounds when she was 17. She lost 25 pounds and maintained a weight of around 120 from age 17 to 23.

Psychological Factors

•Karen was often teased for being overweight as a child; her family referred to her weight as "baby fat."
•Karen's older brother, who was adored by the family, was the center of her life. Karen believed that all of her success was due to him. She was very protective of him.
•Physical affection was not displayed in Karen's home because her mother felt it was not necessary. Friend's described Karen as "starving for love and recognition from her parents."

Social Factors

•American society emphasizes thinness as a sign of beauty.

Sample Multiple-Choice Questions

1. Dorothy weighs 90% of her expected normal weight and has an intense fear of gaining weight. She places undue emphasis on her body weight and shape, which influences her self-esteem. She admitted that she has not had a menstrual cycle for six months now. Dorothy's diagnosis is probably __________.
   a. anorexia nervosa
   b. bulimia nervosa
   c. binge eating disorder
   d. eating disorder not otherwise specified (NOS)

2. Recurrent episodes of binge eating, inappropriate compensatory behaviors to prevent weight gain, and self-evaluation that is unduly influenced by body shape and weight are all symptoms of __________.
   a. anorexia nervosa
   b. bulimia nervosa
   c. binge eating disorder
   d. eating disorder NOS

3. Preliminary data clearly indicate that binge-eating disorder occurs predominantly in individuals who are __________.
   a. obese
   b. average in weight
   c. underweight
   d. impulsive by nature

4. Which of the following statements about familial transmission of eating disorders is TRUE?
   a. Familial transmission of anorexia nervosa occurs through learning and reinforcement only; there is no evidence of a genetic transmission.
   b. Familial transmission of bulimia nervosa occurs through learning and reinforcement only; there is no evidence of a genetic transmission.
   c. Familial transmission of both anorexia nervosa and bulimia nervosa occurs through genetic influences.
   d. Familial transmission of both anorexia nervosa and bulimia nervosa cannot be determined; appropriate studies to detect genetic influences are lacking.

5. Which neurotransmitter plays a key role in regulating mood and eating behaviors?
   a. noradrenaline
   b. serotonin
   c. dopamine
   d. adrenaline

6. Diana rigidly diets and exercises frequently. However, if she gives in to temptation and eats one piece of chocolate, she becomes depressed. She then proceeds to eat the whole box of chocolates along with whatever else she can find in the house. She thinks of herself as a loser after these episodes. This is an example of __________.
   a. carbohydrate craving
   b. purging
   c. the abstinence violation effect
   d. catastrophizing

7. Minuchin and colleagues (1978) identified characteristic patterns of interaction in families of adolescents with anorexia nervosa. Which pattern was supported empirically?
   a. Enmeshment
   b. Overprotectiveness
   c. Rigidity
   d. Conflict avoidant

8. Dr. Zhivago strictly assumes a sociocultural basis to eating disorders. He believes (hypothetically) that if beauty and thinness were a central aspect of masculinity then __________.
   a. the prevalence rates for eating disorders would decrease.
   b. eating disorders would be more prevalent among males than females.
   c. eating disorders would be more prevalent among females than males.
   d. medication would be the most effective treatment for bulimia nervosa.

9. Darcie is 5 feet tall, and her weight has dropped to a dangerous 65 pounds. Her doctor's first priority is to help Darcie gain weight. Which treatment will her doctor most likely choose?
   a. Drug therapy
   b. Family therapy
   c. Behavior modification
   d. Cognitive behavioral therapy

10. Megan is taking antidepressant medication, Carla is in cognitive-behavioral therapy, Valerie is in family therapy and Ann is in psychodynamic therapy. Which patient is getting the most effective treatment for bulimia nervosa?
   a. Ann
   b. Megan
   c. Carla
   d. Valerie

Answer Key

1. d
2. b
3. a
4. c
5. b
6. c
7. a
8. b
9. c
10. c

CHAPTER 12 PERSONALITY DISORDERS

Personality and Personality Disorders

Personality is the more or less stable, characteristic way a person feels and behaves in a wide variety of situations. People are typically able to adapt their behavior to different situations in their lives. Individuals with personality traits that are so exaggerated and inflexible that they distress them or cause problems in their school, work, or interpersonal relationships have a personality disorder. The personality disorders forma second level (Axis II) in the multiaxial system of the DSM-IV. Disorders of Axis I tend to come and go while those of Axis II are longer lasting. The box on page 180 list the DSM-IV General Diagnostic Criteria for Personality Disorder.

Background. The study of personality disorders is usually traced to the concepts of manic sans delire (insanity without delirium) and moral insanity. These refer to the occurrence of wildly inappropriate behaviors in persons whose intellect was otherwise intact. Sigmund Freud and other early psychoanalysts also described a number of character disorders (e.g., melancholic, phobic) and Kurt Schneider identified 10 personality types (e.g., insecure, attention-seeking).

Classification of Personality Disorders. Personality traits are dimensional; people have some quantity of certain characteristics. Personality types are categorical; they are descriptions that center on a few striking features. The DSM-IV classifies personality disorders using a categorical system based on personality types. There are 10 personality disorders, each of which has a few prominent characteristics. In addition, a more detailed set of criteria is given for each personality disorder. To be diagnosed with a personality disorder, a person must show 4 or 5 of these specific criteria.

Description

The DSM-IV groups the personality disorders into three clusters based on descriptive similarities. Table 12.1 on page 382 lists the diagnoses forming each cluster and the descriptive features shared by the disorders in each cluster.

Cluster A: Odd and Eccentric Personality Disorders. Table 12.2 lists the essential features that are specific to each of the three Cluster A diagnoses, which include paranoid, schizoid, and schizotypal. The essential feature of paranoid personality disorder is a pervasive distrust and suspiciousness of others such that their motives are interpreted as malevolent. People with paranoid personality disorder feel slighted by little things and are easily angered by perceived insults that are not apparent to others. The essential features of schizoid personality disorder are a pervasive pattern of detachment from social relationships and a restricted range of emotions in interpersonal settings. Individuals with schizoid personality disorder are reclusive, engaging in solitary activities, can form stable relationships but not close relationships even with family members. Schizotypal personality disorder, is a relatively recent addition. It evolved out of clarifying the boundary between schizophrenia and borderline personality disorder. A schizotypal personality exhibits two sets of qualities: 1) intense discomfort in interpersonal relationships and impaired ability to form close relationships; and 2) cognitive or perceptual distortions and eccentric behaviors. People with schizotypal personality disorder may dress in mismatched clothing, their speech and perception of the world may also be unusual, and they are loners.

Cluster B: Dramatic, Emotional, and Erratic Personality Disorders. Table 12.3 lists the essential features that are specific to each of the three Cluster B diagnoses, which include antisocial, borderline, histrionic, and narcissistic. The essential features of antisocial personality disorder are a pervasive pattern of disregard for and violation of the rights of others occurring since age 15, with evidence of conduct disorder before age 15. This disorder is much more common in males than females (3% and 1%, respectively, display characteristics of antisocial personality disorder). Researchers have been studying an alternative set of criteria based on classic criteria for psychopathy. These criteria emphasize such traits as lack of empathy, glib and superficial charm, egocentricity and inflated sense of self-worth, emotional unresponsiveness and irresponsibility in interpersonal relationships, poor judgment and failure to learn from experience, deceitfulness, and impulsive behavior. Controversy over the overlap between psychopathy and antisocial personality disorder is not resolved by data. Borderline personality disorder is the least distinct of all the personality disorders and has also become one of the most frequently diagnosed personality disorder (about 10% of psychiatric outpatients and 20% of inpatients). The essential features are a pervasive pattern of instability in interpersonal relationships, self-image, and affects, and marked impulsivity. What seems distinct about mood in borderline personality disorder is its reactivity--fluctuation of intense dysphoria, anxiety, and rage within a matter of hours or days. Individuals with borderline personality disorder often act impulsively in self-destructive ways. Table 12.4 on page 385 shows the variety of self-destructive acts of borderline hospital patients. Histrionic personality disorder evolved from the ancient concept of hysteria. The essential feature of this disorder is a pervasive pattern of excessive emotionality and attention seeking in which individuals attempt to gain attention in unusual ways. These individuals are often provocative or sexually seductive, highly impressionable, and shallow about people. The essential features of narcissistic personality disorder are a pervasive pattern of grandiosity, need for admiration, and lack of empathy. Data suggest that more men have narcissistic traits than women, but the full disorder is rarely found among community samples (less than 1%).

Cluster C: Anxious and Fearful Personality Disorders. Table 12.5 lists the essential features that are specific to each of the three Cluster C diagnoses, which include avoidant, dependent, and obsessive-compulsive personality disorders. Avoidant personality disorder was first included in DSM-III. This disorder is characterized by a pervasive pattern of social inhibition, feelings of inadequacy, and hypersensitivity to negative evaluation. These three characteristics are highly intertwined in avoidant people. In contrast to individuals with schizoid personality disorder, those with avoidant personality disorder desire contact with others. Dependent personality disorder is characterized by two interrelated essential features: 1) a pervasive and excessive need to be taken care of; and 2) the submissive and clinging behavior and fears of separation that this need causes. To gain approval and to assure the support of those they depend on, these individuals may voluntarily make unreasonable sacrifices or do mundane and thankless tasks for others. The essential features of obsessive-compulsive personality disorder are preoccupation with orderliness, perfectionism, and mental and interpersonal control, at the expense of flexibility, openness, and efficiency. People with this disorder have inflexible values and are overly conscientious about matters of morality and ethics.

Issues and Problems in Categorizing Personality Disorders

Epidemiology. Research on the prevalence of personality disorders has been hampered by the lack of reliable instruments for assessment. However, recent reviews reported consistent rates cross-nationally. Overall lifetime rate for any personality disorder in community-based samples ranges from about 10 to 13%. In patient samples, prevalence ranged from a low of 2% to a high of 64%. Considerable evidence has also shown that personality disorders overlap with other types of psychological problems, especially Axis I diagnoses.

Reliability. A diagnosis must be consistent and replicable. When two clinicians each conduct diagnostic interviews with patients and show good agreement on the diagnoses they assign, interrater reliability has been established for that interview. If the diagnostic interviews are then repeated on another occasion, using the same set of patients, and the patients are assigned the same diagnoses, good test-retest reliability (or temporal stability) has been established for both the interview and the diagnoses. About 30% of the research on personality disorders has yielded results with poor temporal stability, and most of the research has yielded low test-retest reliability.

Validity. The validity of the current categorical system of diagnosing personality disorders has been challenged repeatedly since it first appeared. First, type or categorical systems assume that individuals in the same category are highly similar, but only 5 of 9 criteria are required for diagnosis of a personality disorder. Second, the assumption that most individuals will clearly fit into a single category is not supported. For example, 85% of individuals who meet the diagnostic criteria for one personality disorder also meet those for at least one other personality disorder, and only 1-2% of those with only one personality disorder could be considered a prototype or good example of the category. Third, the most common diagnosis is the catchall category of personality disorder-not otherwise specified, indicating the difficulty of dividing personality disorders into discrete types. Finally, features of these disorders are hard to define, which results in considerable disagreement in assigning specific diagnoses when different methods are used.

Dimensional Approaches to Describing Personality Disorders. Many researchers of personality disorders believe that it might be better to use a dimensional system in which personality is described using traits rather than diagnostic types. Advantages include: flexibility in describing ever-changing personality problems, solving the difficulty in identifying the objective boundary between personality disorder and normality, and solving the mystery of how personality disorder can be defined as stable patterns representing enduring personality styles yet show such poor test-retest reliability. Because arbitrary diagnostic thresholds are used to decide the presence versus absence of a disorder, the observed unreliability is an artifact, (a research finding that reflects a methodological problem rather than a valid result). DSM-IV has not adopted a dimensional approach because there is not enough evidence to decide which alternative model is best. The approach that is currently the most popular is the five-factor approach to personality which describes five major traits or dimensions: Neuroticism, Extraversion, Agreeableness, Conscientiousness, and Openness to Experience. Table 12.6 on page 395 describes the five factors and illustrates how more extensive sets of dimensions align with these factors and with each other.

Causes

Biological Factors. Four broad dimensions were proposed by Siever and Davis (1991) to account for observed links between biological variables and personality disorder diagnoses. The cognitive/perceptual organization dimension underlies the schizophrenia spectrum, which is a range of disorders including schizophrenia and the Cluster A personality disorders. This view states that difficulty in cognitive/perceptual organization could interfere with the development of satisfying relations between infants and their caregivers and could be starting point for the social awkwardness seen in certain personality disorders. The impulsivity/aggression dimension reflects individual differences in the degree of responsiveness to stimuli, both internal and external. Research has shown that individuals with psychopathic or antisocial personalities are impulsive, have impaired cognitive abilities, fail to learn from negative feedback, and have difficulty delaying gratification. The impulsivity and anxiety experienced by psychopaths may better be viewed as activation of the fight or flight system which is a biological system that responds to unconditioned negative stimuli and directs an organism to action (fleeing or fighting) when threatened. The affective instability dimension is similar to dysregulation in the behavioral activation system. Poor regulation of this system may explain the hyperreactive moodiness of people with Cluster B personality disorders. The anxiety/inhibition dimension is associated with Axis I anxiety disorders and the Cluster C personality disorders. Individuals with marked negative affectivity have an overly strong or active behavioral inhibition system; even mild stimuli represent potential threats. Table 12.7 on page 400 represents different personality trait models that have been proposed to account for individual differences in both normal-range personality and personality disorders.

Psychosocial Factors. A psychosocial approach integrates psychodynamic, social learning and behavioral models. The psychodynamic view is that personality types reflect an internal, intrapsychic organization. Personality disorders result when this internal organization develops in a skewed manner and becomes rigidly maladaptive. Personality disorders may be the result of excessive exposure to stressful and unhealthy life experiences before the person has developed the psychological resources needed to cope with them. The diagnoses of dependent, obsessive-compulsive, and histrionic personality disorders all have their origins in early psychoanalytic theory. Narcissistic and borderline personality disorders have been the focus of psychoanalytic object-relations theory that stresses the influence of early parental relationships in personality development. Attachment theory emphasizes cognitive factors in how children first form their working models of how close relationships operate. Development of personality and personality disorders is based on the quality of the attachment relationship between the child and the primary caregiver. Childhood abuse is an identified risk factor for psychopathology and the best documented psychosocial factor in the development of personality disorder.

Biopsychosocial Approach. Biological factors, such as temperament, set the stage for the range of personality types an individual can develop; environmental factors then interact with basic temperament to shape behavior. For example, periods of rapid social change, or social disintegration, may cause difficulty for individuals with a vulnerability on the cognitive/perceptual dimension. Paris has identified three key points of this model: 1) personality traits or temperaments, which have a strong genetic component, form the basis for personality disorder; 2) negative childhood experiences place individuals at risk for various disorders; and 3) social disintegration places individuals at risk for personality disorder. It is important to assess the extent to which biological, psychological, and social factors contribute to the problems that the individual reports.

Treatment

Pharmacotherapy. The vast majority of drug studies have involved borderline personality disorder. Of the drugs tested (neuroleptics, antidepressants, lithium, carbamazepine, and benzodiazepines), no drug of choice has been identified. Drugs should be used selectively for the short-term treatment of specific problems, rather than for the diagnosis itself. Monoamine oxidase inhibitors (MAOIs), which are used in the treatment of depression, have been found to be effective. Because drugs by themselves do not affect the rigid character pathology found in personality disorder, pharmacotherapy and psychotherapy are often recommended.

Psychodynamic Psychotherapy. Modern psychoanalysts, particularly object-relations theorists, have focused on the patient getting in touch with and accepting the unfulfilled needs of childhood which have resulted in psychopathology. The focus of this approach is primarily on narcissistic and borderline personality disorder with borderline pathology viewed as more serious of the two. Treatment drop-out is common, and intermittent treatment may be the norm for severe personality disorder. The length of time a patient continues in treatment is increased by a positive therapeutic relationship.

Interpersonal Therapy. Benjamin's structural analysis of social behavior (SASB) approach analyzes the interaction of several intrapsychic and interpersonal dimensions to explain behavioral processes involved in personality disorder. This has evolved over 20 years of clinical research, but there are no controlled studies of its effectiveness. Treatment stresses gaining an understanding of one's destructive interaction patterns and developing a more adaptive interpersonal style.

Cognitive Therapy. The core assumption of this approach is that particular errors in thinking are responsible for individuals' behavioral and emotional problems. Cognitive distortions are identified and replaced with more adaptive and realistic cognitions. The approach has incorporated behavioral techniques, such as role-play, imagery, and also incorporates reviewing childhood experiences. Patient drop-out is common and there are no controlled studies evaluating its effectiveness.

Behavior Therapy. This approach has been used in more controlled treatment studies than any other treatment. Most studies involved social skills training and/or graduated exposure for individuals with extreme shyness, social avoidance, and other social deficits. Improvements were sometimes limited to more superficial relationships, and normal levels of functioning and emotional well-being were often not attained. Data support the idea that trait dimensions, rather than diagnoses per se, provide the most useful information for understanding personality disorder.

Dialectic Behavior Therapy (DBT). This is the most promising treatment for severely dysfunctional personality pathology. DBT blends aspects of psychodynamic, client-centered, strategic, interpersonal, cognitive-behavioral, and crisis intervention approaches. It assumes that personality disorder results from multiple causes (i.e., a biopsychosocial approach). The dysfunction that is the core of the personality disorder must interact with what Linehan calls the invalidating environment, which refers to an environment in which significant others negate and/or respond erratically and inappropriately to an individual's private emotional experiences. Sexual abuse is the prototypic invalidating experience for individuals with severe personality disorders. Primary emphasis is placed on acceptance of the individual and his/her experiences and corresponding emphasis on change. DBT consists of a pretreatment (commitment) phase and three treatment stages: 1) stability, connection, and safety; 2) exposure and emotional processing of the past; and 3) synthesis. Data support the theoretical basis of this treatment.

KEY IDEAS AND OBJECTIVES FOR STUDENTS

After reading the chapter, you should be able to answer each of the following questions:

1. When is a personality disorder diagnosed?
2. When did the scientific study of personality disorder begin?
3. What kind of a system is used to diagnose personality disorders?
4. How many personality disorders and how many clusters are used in the DSM-IV?
5. What are the characteristics and specific disorders included in Cluster A?
6. What are the characteristics and specific disorders included in Cluster B?
7. What are the characteristics and specific disorders included in Cluster C?
8. How prevalent are personality disorders and which is the most commonly diagnosed personality disorder?
9. Which disorders occur in combination with personality disorder and how does this affect treatment?
10. How reliable are personality diagnoses and how does agreement vary when different vs same methods are used?

11. How valid are the personality diagnoses? What are the problems with validity?

12. What are trait-dimensional approaches to describing personality disorder? What are the advantages of these systems? What is the five-factor approach to personality?

13. What is the comprehensive psychobiological model for personality disorder proposed by Siever and Davis?

14. What are the primary psychosocial models that have been proposed to help explain the origins of personality disorder? What are the emphasis of object-relations theory and attachment theory?

15. What is the effect of childhood abuse on the development of personality disorder?

16. How does the biopsychosocial approach address the causes of personality disorder; including the related models emphasizing the interactions of temperament and experience in the development of both normal and abnormal personality?

17. Is pharmacotherapy effective in treating personality disorder?

18. What are the characteristics of psychodynamic psychotherapy? Is it effective?

19. What are the characteristics of interpersonal, cognitive, and behavior therapies in the treatment of personality disorder? Are they effective?

20. What is the most promising therapy for severe personality disorder? What is its theoretical and empirical basis? Is it effective?

Personality Disorders in the Movies

1. Fatal Attraction (1987, Paramount Home Video, 120 min) The central character in this film (played by Glenn Close) presents with borderline personality disorder. The instability of her interpersonal relationships and the difficulty she has in maintaining appropriate relationships is presented well in this movie (although students should be made aware of the fact that most persons with borderline personality disorder do not engage in violent behavior towards others). Impulsive actions, suicidal threats and gestures, and self-mutilation are also portrayed. Likewise, periods of apparent normal functioning are evident. Students can identify many of the symptoms and behaviors associated with this personality disorder. Although the ending is very violent and dramatic, students could consider how a pattern of such behavior would affect future ability to form interpersonal relationships.

Questions after watching the movie:

1. Given the text's description of the symptoms and associated behaviors of an individual with borderline personality disorder, how well did the movie do in presenting an accurate portrayal of this disorder? What "errors" (including errors of omission and commission) were made?

2. How did the film deal with the etiology of this disorder? What were the major consistencies (or inconsistencies) with contemporary theories?

3. Are there any other personality disorders which the central character displayed? What symptoms or behaviors would lead you to believe that the central character displayed additional personality disorders?

4. Although the film did not deal with the issue of treatment, what treatments would you recommend for this character?

5. If you were to be a consultant on a "remake" of this film, what advice would you give the director to help make the symptoms, etiology, and treatment more contemporary?

2. Natural Born Killers (1994, Warner, 118 min) The two characters in this movie display characteristics of antisocial personality disorder and/or psychopathy. The characters display aggressive, homicidal behaviors, lack of empathy, superficial charm, egocentricity, inflated self-worth, emotional unresponsiveness, deceitfulness, and impulsive behavior. Social norms are repeatedly violated, the safety of others is disregarded, and the characters show little to no remorse for their actions. In addition to identifying the symptoms and behaviors associated with this personality disorder, students may consider whether treatment, incarceration, or the death penalty is most appropriate for those with severely antisocial behaviors.

Questions after watching the movie:

1. Given the text's description of the symptoms and behaviors associated with antisocial personality disorder (and psychopathy), how well did this movie do in presenting an accurate portrayal of this disorder? Were there differences in the way in which the male and female characters displayed antisocial characteristics? What "errors" (including errors of omission and commission) were made?

2. How did the film deal with the etiology of this disorder? What were the major consistencies (or inconsistencies) with contemporary theories?

3. Are there any other personality disorders which the central characters displayed (e.g., narcissistic, histrionic)? What behaviors would lead you to believe that the two characters displayed these disorders?

4. What treatment (other than legal consequences) was used in this film? What treatments would you recommend for these individuals?

5. If you were to be a consultant for a "remake" of this film, what advice would you give the director to help make the symptoms, etiology, and treatment more contemporary?

Using Case Studies in Abnormal Psychology by Meyer & Osborne:
The Personality Disorders

Chapter 11 in the casebook presents case material on personality disorders with specific information on two disorders. Histrionic personality disorder is portrayed in the case of Hilde. Antisocial personality disorder is portrayed in the case of Theodore Bundy, a serial killer who was executed for his crimes. Each case focuses on applying the diagnostic criteria of each disorder to the behaviors and characteristics displayed, exploring events in childhood and in their respective families which may have contributed to the development of the personality disorders, and in the case of Hilde, treatment is described.

Case Comparisons

The Histrionic Personality Disorder: The Case of Hilde. Hilde, a middle-aged woman, initially presented with somatic complaints, depression and marital difficulties. In the course of the initial sessions, Hilde displayed many of the characteristics of histrionic personality disorder. The characteristics of this personality disorder are presented on page 386 of the text. Provide a summary of the specific characteristics of Hilde that support this diagnosis. Are any of the criteria questionable? Did Hilde display any characteristics of additional personality disorders? Support your answer with specific examples. What factors may have contributed to the development of this disorder for Hilde? Which theoretical models are linked to these factors? What treatment options were considered? Which was used?

Antisocial Personality Disorder: The Case of Theodore Bundy. The diagnostic criteria for antisocial personality disorder and psychopathy are presented on pages 383-384 of your text. Provide a summary of the specific characteristics of Ted that support the diagnosis using each of the criteria. Are any of the criteria questionable? Did Ted meet criteria for any other personality disorder? What factors may have led to the development of this problem? Which theoretical models are linked to these factors? Which treatments would be considered if Ted had not been executed? (It might also be useful to ask students to consider the problems with retrospective reports of those who knew Ted as a child who were interviewed after he was a convicted killer.)

Integrating Perspectives
A Biopsychosocial Model

The Case of Hilde

Biological Factors

- Hilde was extremely beautiful.

Psychological Factors

- Hilde appeared to have great intellectual potential, but her parents provided no encouragement. In fact, her parents made fun of individuals whom they called 'Intellectual snobs."
- Hilde learned early that she could avoid punishment at home by using her charms with her parents.

Social Factors

- Hilde was raised as a prized child of a moderately wealthy family.

Sample Multiple-Choice Questions

1. A(n) _______ is a more or less stable, characteristic way a person feels and behaves in a wide variety of situations.
   a. ego
   b. personality
   c. state
   d. superego

2. Herb is a very organized person. This description of Herb is an example of a personality _______.
   a. cluster
   b. type
   c. trait
   d. state

3. A ________ is a group of personality disorders which share descriptive characteristics.
   a. prototype
   b. trait
   c. type
   d. cluster

4. Debbie is an unmarried, forty-two year-old data entry clerk. Debbie prefers to engage in solitary activities, such as reading and sewing, when she is not working. Debbie sees her family about twice a year, but does not have close relationships with family members. Although Debbie's job requires little social interaction with others, when Debbie interacts with coworkers, her coworkers often describe Debbie as being "cold and distant." Debbie's personality traits can best be described as ________.
   a. dependent
   b. schizoid
   c. antisocial
   d. obsessive-compulsive

5. Which of the following personality disorders is best characterized by social inhibition, feelings of inadequacy, and extreme sensitivity to negative remarks?
   a. Schizoid
   b. Schizotypal
   c. Dependent
   d. Avoidant

6. A technician uses a diagnostic interview with a patient while two doctors observe. Dr. Benning gave the diagnosis of avoidant personality disorder and Dr. Wilkins gave the diagnosis of dependent personality disorder. The diagnostic interview appears to have poor _______.
   a. test-retest reliability
   b. interrater reliability
   c. test-retest validity
   d. interrater validity

7. Betty has been diagnosed with only one personality disorder. She meets all of the diagnostic criteria for this personality disorder. She is considered the perfect example of how someone with this personality disorder behaves. Betty is an example of a _______.
   a. diagnostic model
   b. criterion model
   c. prototype
   d. categotype

8. Lloyd's mother is schizophrenic. Lloyd has been diagnosed with schizotypal personality disorder. Lloyd shows attentional abnormalities. It is believed that these attentional abnormalities are connected to Lloyd's detachment from others. Which one of Siever and Davis' dimensions would most likely account for the link between biological variables and Lloyd's personality disorder?
   a. impulsivity/aggression
   b. anxiety/inhibition
   c. affective instability
   d. cognitive/perceptual organization

9. Siever and Davis relate the _______ dimension to Axis I anxiety disorders and the Axis II, Cluster C personality disorders.
   a. cognitive/perceptual organization
   b. impulsivity/aggression
   c. affective instability
   d. anxiety/inhibition

10. Greg has been diagnosed with dependent personality disorder. Greg's therapist says that Greg's personality disorder reflects Greg's internal, intrapsychic organization. Greg's therapist says that Greg's personality disorder developed because as a child Greg's father left the family. Greg's therapist says that as a result Greg felt he had to try and please everyone so that he would not be left again. Greg's therapist most likely adheres to the _______ model.
    a. cognitive
    b. behavioral
    c. psychodynamic
    d. humanistic

Answer Key

1. b
2. c
3. d
4. b
5. d
6. b
7. c
8. d
9. d
10. c

CHAPTER 13 SCHIZOPHRENIA

This chapter introduces disorders of psychosis (involving loss of touch with reality; involving delusions, hallucinations, and disorganized speech/behavior. The chapter opens with the case of John Nash, winner of the 1994 Nobel Prize in Economics and traces the effects of schizophrenia on his life.

Description

Emil Kraeplin first described schizophrenia, under the term dementia praecox ("premature dementia"). He initially identified three subtypes (catatonia, hebephrenia, and paranoia), later adding Bleuler's simple schizophrenia. Kraeplin believed that continual deterioration in the brain was the cause of schizophrenia, which began in early adolescence and had a chronic course. Modern views differ from Kraeplin's. While most hospital admissions occur in late adolescence and early adulthood, the first schizophrenic episode can occur at almost point in life. Late-onset individuals may have married, held jobs and maintained multiple social interactions. Individuals often suffer more than one serious episode, but may also have long symptom-free periods. Eugen Bleuler coined the term schizophrenia. He differed from Kraeplin in that he believed that early onset was not necessary and that mental deterioration was not inevitable. He also, however, thought that biological factors were important in the development of schizophrenia, which interacted with environmental stress to produce the disorder. Bleuler focused on what he believed to be the underlying feature of schizophrenia - a loosening of associations between thoughts and feelings. Individuals with schizophrenia experience a splitting of thoughts and feelings, but do NOT experience split personalities (e.g., dissociative identity disorder).

Prevalence. Lifetime prevalence for schizophrenia is only about 1%. However, people are incapacitated and are more likely to require hospitalization than those with other serious disorders. Onset is usually between ages 16 and 25; onset after age 35 is uncommon. An equal number of males and females develop the disorder; however, males tend to develop the disorder during their early- to mid-20s while females tend to develop the disorder during the late-20s. Thus, males are first hospitalized at an earlier age than are females. Reasons for these gender differences are explored in Thinking About Gender Issues: Why Do Males Have Earlier Ages of Onset? on page 414. Symptoms tend to decrease with increasing age, with few symptoms of the disorder evident after age 50. This contrasts with earlier theories that schizophrenia is a progressive disorder. Harding and colleagues conducted a long-term (25 years) followup study of schizophrenic patients. Only half of the persons regularly took antipsychotic medication and 45% did not exhibit any symptoms of schizophrenia. Two-thirds were functioning very well. The majority were meeting daily living needs, had weekly social activities, and had not been recently hospitalized. These results indicate that while some individuals experience chronic, severe impairment, others do not continue to deteriorate and may even improve their functioning. Regional differences in long-term outcome have led some to propose that recovery is related to the level of care received from the community.

Definition and Symptoms. The DSM-IV criteria for schizophrenia are presented on page 416. At least two of the following symptoms must be present for at least 6 months and have a marked effect on social and work relations: 1) delusions, 2) hallucinations, 3) disorganized speech, 4) grossly disorganized or catatonic behavior, and 5) negative symptoms. If delusions are bizarre or hallucinations consist of a running commentary of the person's thoughts or behaviors, only one symptom is required for diagnosis. If at least two voices converse with one another, this is sufficient for the diagnosis. Because no single psychotic symptom must be present to meet criteria, there can be considerable variability among those with the diagnosis. It is important to distinguish schizophrenia from other disorders, such as bipolar disorders or substance abuse.

Symptoms of schizophrenia can be classified into positive and negative symptoms. Positive symptoms are behaviors and feelings normally not present in the general population; these include delusions, hallucinations, disorganized speech, and disorganized and catatonic behavior. Delusions are false beliefs or unusual misrepresentations of reality. Delusions of persecution are characterized by a clear theme that others are out to get the individual. These are present in about 65% of patients with schizophrenia. Delusions of grandeur are characterized by a belief that the individual is a highly important person (e.g., Jesus Christ, Elvis Presley); beliefs that the individual has special powers are also included in this category. Delusions of control involve a belief that one's thoughts or actions are controlled by external factors, such as persons or forces from another planet. Delusions of romance (erotomania) are false beliefs that someone is in love with or romantically involved with the individual. John Hinckley's obsession with Jodie Foster is described to illustrate this characteristic. Men with schizophrenia are least likely to exhibit delusions of romance. Foreign-born Americans are most prone to paranoid delusions, and high SES level persons with schizophrenia are most likely to have delusions of grandeur. While delusions are not specific to schizophrenia, the more bizarre the delusions the more characteristic they are of schizophrenia.

Hallucinations are sensory experiences in the absence of external environmental stimulation. Auditory and visual hallucinations are the most common, with 70% of schizophrenic individuals reporting auditory hallucinations and 25% reporting visual hallucinations (10% report other hallucinations). Hallucinations tend to worsen with social isolation. Research suggests that schizophrenic patients are unable to distinguish between inner speech and reality. Involvement in activities may serve as a distracter to hallucinations, which are reported less frequently by individuals actively involved in tasks. Disorganized speech occurs when a person's speech is incomprehensible or remotely related to the topic of conversation. Derailment occurs when a person moves from one topic to another without any natural transitions. Tangentiality occurs when a person responds in a manner that seems unrelated to the prompt or question of another person. Illogicality refers to drawing conclusions that don't follow from what was just said. Disorganized speech is a symptom of schizophrenia only when 1) the disorganization is severe enough to make effective communication nearly impossible and 2) if the disorganized speech occurs in conjunction with another of the five DSM symptoms. The final positive symptom of schizophrenia is grossly disorganized behavior, which involves an inability to persist in goal-directed behavior, or inappropriate behavior in public. Catatonic behavior involves marked motor abnormalities such as bizarre postures, purposeless motor activity, and extreme degree of unawareness.

Negative symptoms include three deficits: 1) flat or blunted affect, 2) little speech (alogia), and 3) lack of drive, or avolition. Flat affect refers to lack of emotional expressiveness in gesture, facial expression, and voice tone, and is apparent in about 50% of schizophrenic persons. Alogia refers to poverty of speech in which the individual talks very little and/or gives brief, empty replies to questions. Avolition involves the inability to begin and sustain goal-directed activity and the expression of little or no interest in activities. Persons with high levels of negative symptoms have more cognitive deficits, less education, lower intelligence, and greater problems in social functioning than those with primarily positive symptoms. They are less responsive to medication and are associated with poorer outcome. Anhedonia, or the inability to experience pleasure in physical (eating, drinking, sexual activities) or social contact is often associated with schizophrenia, but is not a criteria for the disorder.

Phases and Types of Schizophrenia. Individuals differ with regard to their functioning prior to the first episode of schizophrenic symptoms. Some were well-adjusted socially and personally, while others display problems in childhood and adolescence (social withdrawal and lack of responsiveness, and hyperactivity, conduct problems, and impulsive behavior). Schizophrenia is characterized by different phases in which symptoms and functioning vary considerably. The prodromal phase refers to the period immediately before significant symptoms of schizophrenia are evident. During this phase, the person withdraws socially, displays poor grooming, has difficulty communicating, shows lack of initiative, and has some bizarre thoughts. Others often notice a personality change during this phase. The active or acute phase follows the prodromal phase and is characterized by psychotic symptoms (delusions, hallucinations, loose associations, and unusual motor behavior). This phase may be associated with a stressful event. The residual phase follows the active phase and is similar to the prodromal phase; it is characterized by social withdrawal, inactivity, and bizarre thoughts. Negative symptoms are often prominent during this phase, along with impaired social and vocational functioning.

There are five types of schizophrenia. The catatonic type is characterized by unusual patterns of motor activity, such as rigid postures and stupor or trancelike states. Speech disturbances such as repetitive chatter or mutism are common with this type. Onset is usually sudden with this type, which is much less common today than during the 1950s. The disorganized type is characterized by verbal incoherence, grossly disorganized behavior, marked loosening of associations, and inappropriate affect. These individuals do not display elaborate sets of delusions; their delusions and hallucinations are not usually organized around a particular theme. They may also display unusual mannerisms (e.g., grimacing), extreme social withdrawal and social impairment. Onset is usually early in life and significant remission or recovery is rare. The paranoid type individual is preoccupied with one or more sets of delusions organized around one or more central themes. They may also have hallucinations with a single theme. They don't have grossly inappropriate affect or disorganized behavior, but do display extreme motor symptoms characteristic of the catatonic type. They may show anger and occasionally become violent. If delusions are intense and they fear physical harm, they may become severely anxious and panic. Prognosis for these individuals is much better than for other types. The undifferentiated type person displays delusions, hallucinations, and incoherence, but do not meet the criteria for any of the other types. Residual-type schizophrenia usually occurs after prominent delusions, hallucinations, or formal thought disorder have stopped; individuals still speak very little, show little affect, have little to no motivation, and experience some irregular beliefs.

Causes

Schizophrenia appears to have a genetic basis, but environmental factors contribute to the disorder. Thus, an interactive model fits this disorder.

Biological Factors. Three types of biological factors appear to be important in the development of schizophrenia. Genetic predisposition to schizophrenia is supported by family and twin studies; a vulnerability to the disease may be inherited (rather than the disorder itself). First-degree relatives of schizophrenic persons have approximately a 5% chance of becoming schizophrenic, compared to a 0.5% chance in relatives of a normal control sample. This risk is 10 times greater for family members of schizophrenic individuals than for controls. Twin studies have yielded consistent results. The concordance rate for monozygotic/identical twins is 50%, while it is only 15 to 20 percent for dizygotic/fraternal twins. Although results vary somewhat depending on the stringency of the definition for inclusion, the more severe the symptoms in the schizophrenic twin, the greater likelihood that the co-twin is also schizophrenic. Adoption studies provide similar results which strongly indicate that genetic factors are key in the development of schizophrenia. Table 13.1 on page 426 and Figure 13.2 on page 427 illustrate the relationship between genetics and schizophrenia. A multifactorial polygenic model, which is an etiological model that proposes that many genes interact with environmental influences to lead to a psychiatric disorder, is useful in explaining schizophrenia. It estimates that genetic influences contribute 60-70%, with environmental influences accounting for the remaining 30-40% of the cause. Thus, environmental factors may be critical for those at genetic risk for the disorder.

Brain dysfunction has also been investigated as a cause of schizophrenia. Magnetic resonance imaging (MRI) focuses on the brain structure, and schizophrenic individuals have been shown to have enlarged ventricles. The degree of enlargement is correlated with cognitive impairment; decreased brain volume is related to the severity of hallucinations, disorganized speech (in the temporal region), and with blunted affect and lack of motivation (frontal area). Positron-emission tomographic (PET) scans assess bloodflow in the brain and demonstrate brain function. Schizophrenic persons have abnormally low activity in their frontal lobes, which control executive planning. Neuropsychological tests also assess brain function. A study by Cannon et al. found that level of neuropsychological impairment was greater in schizophrenic individuals, was intermediate in siblings of the schizophrenic individuals, and lowest in a matched control group. Results suggest that frontal and temporal lobe dysfunction is related to schizophrenia. Additional support for frontal lobe dysfunction comes from research demonstrating that schizophrenic persons have trouble with smooth-pursuit eye-tracking tasks (visually following a continuously moving target). Dysfunction on these tasks has been found to be the best biological indicator of genetic liability to develop schizophrenia.

Biochemical abnormalities have been examined as causes of the disorder. Antipsychotic medications often cause side effects involving Parkinsonian movements. Since Parkinsonism was related to abnormally low levels of dopamine, it was hypothesized that schizophrenia was due to excess dopamine. Antipsychotic medications were thought to reduce hallucinations by reducing dopamine levels (which led to Parkinsonian movements). The dopamine hypothesis generated much research and has some validity. However, schizophrenic patients and nonschizophrenic controls have not been found to differ in dopamine levels. Also, antipsychotic medications affect multiple neurotransmitters, only one of which is dopamine. Serotonin and norepinephrine have been identified as potentially important; however, research has yielded conflicting data.

Psychological Factors. During the 1960s research emphasized family stress and communication problems as risk factors for schizophrenia. Laing proposed that schizophrenia develops when people retreat as a way of coping with overwhelming stress. Szasz proposed that schizophrenia was a function of society's attempt to control unusual or unacceptable behavior. These views did not significantly alter mainstream views of schizophrenia; however, they were consistent with efforts to examine the social context in which mental illness occurs. Recent life events may affect the onset and recurrence of schizophrenic episodes. Communication abnormalities in families of persons with schizophrenia where thought to cause the disorder. The double-bind hypothesis proposed that contradictory messages from another person (i.e., the parent) would cause stress in a child, which would then lead to schizophrenia. Research did not support this hypothesis. Families of schizophrenic persons, however, do demonstrate communication deviance, a rejecting or indifferent parental style, and a detached family environment. It is impossible to determine whether these characteristics are the cause of schizophrenia and/or the result of living with a family member who was preschizophrenic and perhaps deviant as a child. Thus, there is no evidence that parental factors cause schizophrenia. High-risk studies follow children at risk for developing schizophrenia (i.e., one parent is schizophrenic) to determine differences between those who develop the disorder and those who do not. Subjects who became schizophrenic were characterized by the following: mothers with more severe schizophrenia; more frequent separation from parents and placement in children's homes; greater perinatal birth difficulties; higher teacher ratings of aggressiveness and becoming easily angered; and higher autonomic arousal levels, especially for those developing hallucinations and delusions. Marital discord was not a factor, but viral infections during pregnancy and other birth traumas were associated with developing schizophrenia.

Social Class Factors. Epidemiological studies have consistently found higher rates of mental illness among lower social classes. Table 13.2 on page 434 presents the prevalence of schizophrenia by social class. The greater prevalence has been explained by two different hypotheses. The social causation hypothesis proposes that factors associated with being a member of a lower SES class may contribute to the development of schizophrenia. Thus, poor prenatal care, poor nutrition, unequal access to early treatment, and relatively lower family, social and medical support increase the risk of schizophrenia. The social selection hypothesis states that persons genetically predisposed to schizophrenia drift downward to lower SES classes. Research has yielded conflicting support for these two hypotheses, although one study suggests that social selection may be a stronger contributor than socioeconomic class.

Eisenberg applied an interactive model, the diathesis-stress model, which proposed that preexisting vulnerability (genetic, biological, and/or psychological vulnerability, or the diathesis) interacts with stress (poverty, severe criticism from family members) to cause schizophrenia.

The biopsychosocial model is broader in that biological, psychological, and social variables can be incorporated. In addition, individual differences in severity and course of the disorder can be explained by this model. The Integrating Perspectives: A Biopsychosocial Model box on page 437 outlines biological, psychological and social factors that may lead to schizophrenia and examines a case to illustrate the model.

Family Variables. Family variables (in conjunction with medication compliance) are powerful predictors of good outcome in schizophrenic individuals. Families characterized by hostility, dominance, and high levels of criticism and overinvolvement with the schizophrenic individual are labeled high expressed emotion (or high EE) families. High EE has been linked to higher relapse in patients discharged from the hospital. It is unclear, however, if high EE occurs because patients are more disturbed at the time of discharge, or whether high EE families are less able to care for their schizophrenic relatives.

Treatment

Prior to the 1960s, treatment involved long-term hospitalization (often life-long), insulin injections, prefrontal leukotomy (removal of portion of frontal lobe), ECT, and psychoanalysis. The discovery of neuroleptic medications in the 1950s, emphasis on social causes of schizophrenia in the 1960s, and the rise of community psychology and psychiatry in the 1970s all contributed to the deinstitutionalization movement of the 1960s and 1970s. This movement involved marked reductions in the number of persons in public psychiatric hospitals; patients were returned to their home communities where it was thought that they would be able to function. However, by the 1980s concern was raised that this movement was directly linked to the rising numbers of homeless persons in large metropolitan areas. Effective community services are lacking and/or inadequate for many persons.

Pharmacological Treatment. Chlorpromazine was initially noted to produce a calming effect in patients undergoing surgery. When it was administered to schizophrenic patients, it was found to produce a similar calming effect, but also to significantly reduce hallucinations and delusions. Antipsychotic medications reduce psychotic symptoms, but do not cure or eliminate the disorder. Other medications include chlorpromazine (Thorazine) and haloperidol (Haldol). New antipsychotic medications include clozapine (Clozaril) and risperidone (Risperdal), which affect serotonin receptors. These are effective for people who do not respond to other antipsychotic medications; also, they do not significantly affect motor functioning and have the added benefit of reducing negative symptoms. Clozaril has sedating effects and may cause agranulocytosis, a life-threatening condition in which white blood cell count is reduced. Therefore, the drug must be closely monitored, which can raise the cost to $10,000 per year. Risperdal improves positive and negative symptoms, and has a low rate of motor side effects; side effects include insomnia, agitation and headache. It is considered one of the first choices for treatment. Antipsychotic medications have demonstrated long-term efficacy: relapse and rehospitalization are reduced significantly with medication. However, side effects can be serious. Tardive dyskinesia is a largely irreversible side effect characterized by involuntary lip smacking, tongue movements, and chin wagging. It develops in approximately 20-25% of the population taking antipsychotic medication. Low, or intermittent doses may prevent or diminish the side effect. Approximately 30% of schizophrenic individuals still relapse with medication, which has hastened the search for new, more effective drugs with reduced side effects.

Psychological Treatment. Although Freud viewed schizophrenia as largely organic, Harry Stack Sullivan applied a modified version of psychodynamic therapy to schizophrenia. He viewed schizophrenics' symptoms as a defense to keep distance from others who might damage their already low self-esteem. Feelings of inferiority, loneliness, and failure in living caused anxiety, which could be alleviated by therapy aimed at regressing or returning patients to early childhood experiences to address anxieties at critical points in life. Psychodynamic therapists today increasingly focus on current interpersonal relationship patterns, usually as an adjunct to medication. Although research does not support the efficacy of psychodynamic treatment, it continues to be a central component of many programs. Milieu therapy focuses on the responsibilities of patients to seek employment, care for themselves, and participate in social activities. Self-care, self-management of ward activities, and group norms for appropriate ward behavior are emphasized. Social learning approaches to therapy use reinforcement principles to promote behavior change. Patients earn tokens for privileges (e.g., weekend passes) for appropriate behavior and dress, and participation in group activities. Research has shown that a milieu program and a social learning program were both superior in improving interpersonal skills, self-care and ward activities compared to routine ward care. Despite these results, social learning programs are used infrequently, perhaps because of the time and effort required of staff, and the emphasis on short-term hospitalization and outpatient care. Social skills training using behavioral techniques is promising. Family therapy has been used to help families develop specific techniques they could use at home to deal with the schizophrenic person's difficulties. Family therapy, both alone and in combination with individual therapy for the schizophrenic individual, effectively reduces relapse.

Combined Pharmacological, Psychological, and Social Interventions. Assertive case management is an approach involving multiple systems of intervention, medication, psychological services, and social services to coordinate delivery of services to patients in their communities and homes. Continuous, reliable, extensive support is provided to help the individual live successfully in the community. A consumer movement is underway to share techniques to manage symptoms and de-stigmatize mental illness.

KEY IDEAS AND OBJECTIVES FOR STUDENTS

After reading the chapter, you should be able to answer each of the following questions:

1. When did the study of schizophrenia begin? What were the contributions Emil Kraeplin and Eugen Bleuler?

2. What is the prevalence of schizophrenia and how does it differ among males and females? How does age of onset vary?

3. How do symptoms and outcome vary with age, geographic location, urban vs rural location, and by SES level?

4. What are the characteristics and symptoms of schizophrenia?

5. What are the positive symptoms of schizophrenia? What are the negative symptoms?

6. What are the phases of schizophrenia? How do the phases differ in terms of positive and negative symptoms?

7. What are the five types of schizophrenia?

8. What is the evidence for familial transmission of schizophrenia?

9. Biological research with MRIs and PET scans has shown that people with schizophrenia have structural and functional brain abnormalities, especially in the frontal and temporal areas.

10. How are birth trauma and viral infections related to the development of schizophrenia?

11. What are the theories about the role of biochemical abnormalities in the development of schizophrenia? Is there support for these theories?

12. How does communication differ in the families of people with schizophrenia? How does this affect the development of schizophrenia in high-risk individuals?

13. What is the relationship between the prevalence of schizophrenia and SES, and how is this related to the development of schizophrenia?

14. What is the biopsychosocial models of schizophrenia? What factors are emphasized with this model?

15. What is expressed emotion (EE) and how is this related relapse in discharged schizophrenic patients?

16. What are the effects of antipsychotic drugs and how are they related to deinstitutionalization?

17. What are the side effects and limitations of antipsychotic drugs? What are the advantages of the more recently developed antipsychotic medications?

18. What is the focus of psychodynamic treatments for schizophrenia? Are they effective?

19. What are the characteristics of milieu therapy and social learning therapy for schizophrenia? Are they effective?

20. How are social skills training and family therapy used in the treatment of schizophrenia? Are they effective?

21. What is assertive case management and is it effective in the treatment of schizophrenia?

Schizophrenia in the Movies

1. Awakenings (1990, Columbia TriStar, 120 min) This movie portrays patients who contracted encephalitis and subsequently developed severe cognitive and emotional impairments. While the patients do not have schizophrenia, they display many of the symptoms of the disorder, including catatonia. Antipsychotic medications were initially very effective; however, side effects, including tardive dyskinesia, developed. Robert DeNiro's portrayal of tardive dyskinesia is very realistic and can give students an appreciation for the severity of this side effect.

Questions after watching the movie:

1. What symptoms of schizophrenia were illustrated in this movie? (Be sure to note that the patients in this movie did not have schizophrenia.)

2. What was the etiology of these symptoms? Does this provide any support for a brain dysfunction model of schizophrenia?

3. Would the risk of tardive dyskinesia outweigh the benefits of antipsychotic medication? Who should be the one to decide this?

2. The Fisher King (1991, Columbia TriStar, 137 min) This film portrays Robin Williams as an individual with schizophrenia. Onset occurred following a traumatic event (observing the murder of his wife). Hallucinations are vividly illustrated in this movie, which uses a psychodynamic approach in the interpretation of the thematic content of the hallucinations and delusions. This film can also serve to illustrate homelessness in the mentally ill and how one could judge what is acceptable and unacceptable functioning.

Questions after watching the film:

1. Given the text's description of the symptoms and associated behaviors of schizophrenia, how well did the movie do in presenting an accurate portrayal of this disorder? Can you determine which subtype of schizophrenia was displayed? What "errors" (including errors of omission and commission) were made?

2. How did the film deal with the etiology of this disorder? What were the major consistencies (or inconsistencies) with contemporary theories?

3. What treatment was used in this film? What treatments would you recommend for this individual?

4. If you were to be a consultant for a "remake" of this film, what advice would you give the director to help make the symptoms, etiology, and treatment more contemporary?

Using Case Studies in Abnormal Psychology by Meyer & Osborne:
The Schizophrenic and Delusional (or Paranoid) Disorders

Chapter 6 in the casebook presents three cases to illustrate schizophrenia. Undifferentiated schizophrenia is illustrated in the case of Sally. Paranoid schizophrenia is illustrated in the case of Daniel Paul Schreber, whose analysis by Freud and subsequent book made him famous. Lastly, the case of Lloyd is presented to demonstrate the differences between paranoid schizophrenia and paranoid personality disorder. Premorbid factors, use of antipsychotic medication, etiology, and treatment are addressed in this chapter.

Case Comparisons

Undifferentiated Schizophrenia: The Case of Sally. Sally developed schizophrenia relatively early in life (during college), although her premorbid functioning (functioning during the prodromal phase) was clearly impaired. During the active phase, Sally displayed many of the characteristics of schizophrenia. The DSM criteria for schizophrenia are presented on page 416 of your text. Provide a summary of the specific characteristics of Sally that support this diagnosis. Are any of the criteria questionable? Did Sally display any of the characteristics of the other subtypes of schizophrenia? Support your answers with specific examples. What factors may have contributed to the development of schizophrenia for Sally? Which theoretical models are linked to these factors? What treatments options were considered? How could treatment been more effective for Sally?

Paranoid Schizophrenia: The Case of Daniel Paul Schreber. The diagnostic criteria for schizophrenia are presented on page 416 of your text. Provide a summary of the specific characteristics of Daniel that support this diagnosis using each of the criteria. Are any of the criteria questionable? Did Daniel display any of the characteristics of the other subtypes of schizophrenia? The casebook presents a psychodynamic model. What other theoretical models could be applied to this case? What treatment would be recommended today for Daniel?

Paranoid Personality Disorder: The Case of Lloyd. This case illustrates the personality disorder which is similar to paranoid schizophrenia. The criteria for paranoid personality disorder are presented on pages 381-382. Provide a summary of the characteristics of paranoid personality disorder displayed by Lloyd. Did he display any of the criteria for schizophrenia? Support your answers with specific examples. A psychodynamic model is also used for this case. Compare and contrast the factors which appear to have led to paranoid personality disorder in Lloyd with those associated with paranoid schizophrenia in Daniel. What are the primary distinctions between these two disorders?

Integrating Perspectives
A Biopsychosocial Model

The Case of Sally

Biological Factors

•Sally's mother continued to smoke two packs of cigarettes a day during pregnancy. Early on, Sally had respiratory trouble that resulted in her turning blue for several moments.
•Sally's maternal grandfather was seen by some as "eccentric" and by others as "nuts." He had developed a number of unique religious beliefs.
•Sally was slow to develop. She walked and talked late.

Psychological Factors

•Sally's parents were in constant conflict. They separated briefly when she was 10, but conflict remained.
•Sally was an only child. Her mother had miscarried twice and was encouraged to not try to have other children.
•Sally had above average intelligence, but her performance was below average. She often slipped into fantasy behavior. Her teacher once said that she was "just a bit off center."

Social Factors

•Social factors may have played less of a role, however, her unusual behaviors were not well received at school. Many of her college roommates moved out when they observed her talking to herself.

Sample Multiple-Choice Questions

1. The term "psychotic" usually refers to ________ and ________.
   a. anxiety and depression
   b. hallucinations and delusions
   c. generalized anxiety disorder and social phobia
   d. catatonia and hebephrenia

2. The symptomatology of schizophrenia tends to ________ with age.
   a. stay the same
   b. increase
   c. decrease
   d. get worse

3. Anna believes the president is in love with her and often hears voices which she believes to be from secret service men sent to protect her. When she discusses her special romance, she does not smile and has a very solemn facial expression. She speaks in a monotonous, dull tone. Anna is exhibiting the negative symptom of ________.
   a. alogia
   b. avolition
   c. blunted affect
   d. erotomania

4. Ruth is usually angry and sometimes violent when agitated. She is convinced that the CIA is out to get her. She prefers to be hospitalized because she feels safe there. Ruth is diagnosed with ________ type of schizophrenia.
   a. disorganized
   b. undifferentiated
   c. paranoid
   d. catatonic

5. Which model is currently used to subtype schizophrenia?
   a. A single disease leads to diverse manifestations or symptoms, as with multiple sclerosis.
   b. Varied disorders or diseases lead to schizophrenia by different processes as with mental retardation.
   c. Specific symptom clusters within schizophrenia come together in different ways in different patients.
   d. Individuals with schizophrenia are grouped by physiological or neurological markers.

6. Some individuals with schizophrenia may have developed the disorder as the result of ________.
   a. complications during pregnancy
   b. birth complications
   c. prenatal exposure to influenza or other viruses
   d. all of the above

7. While the research on communication patterns in families of schizophrenic patients cannot determine that families cause schizophrenia, some characteristics have been noted. This research has found that families of schizophrenic patients display all of the following EXCEPT ________.
   a. communication deviance
   b. rejecting or indifferent parental style
   c. detached family environment
   d. double-bind communication

8. If you feared developing schizophrenia, which of the following would you NOT need to avoid?
   a. living in an urban area
   b. living an underdeveloped country
   c. living in a very poor household
   d. living in a highly emotionally-expressive family filled with conflict

9. Which of the following statements about drug treatment for schizophrenia is FALSE?
   a. It is regarded as the single most effective treatment for schizophrenia.
   b. Antipsychotics reduce negative symptoms, but have little impact on positive symptoms of schizophrenia.
   c. Antipsychotic medication often prevents relapse or reentry into the hospital.
   d. The development of antipsychotic medications led to the deinstitutionalization movement.

10. Two new medications, ________ and ________, are effective in the treatment of schizophrenia and have the advantage of fewer side effects than other antipsychotic medications.
   a. chlorpromazine, thorazine
   b. stellazine, haldol
   c. wellbutrin, prozac
   d. clozapine, resperidone

Answer Key

1. b
2. c
3. c
4. c
5. c
6. d
7. d
8. b
9. b
10. d

CHAPTER 14 CHILDHOOD DISORDERS

This chapter covers the majority of childhood disorders. An overview of childhood disorders introduces the topic. Oppositional defiant disorder, conduct disorder, attention-deficit/hyperactivity disorder, anxiety disorders, enuresis, learning disorders, and childhood depression are then presented.

Perspectives on Childhood Disorders

Prior to 1900, children were viewed as downward extensions of adults, and little treatment was provided. Leightner Witmer founded the first clinic for treatment of children in 1898, and Freud's account of Little Hans in 1909 was the first involving psychoanalytic treatment of a child. The Healy School for juvenile delinquents was founded in 1909. These events led to the development of treatment programs for children during the 1930s and 1950s, through child guidance clinics, and a growing recognition that children's problems differed distinctly from those of adults. During the 1970s graduate degrees in clinical child psychology were developed and journals were established which were devoted solely to publication of papers regarding childhood disorders. The DSM-II had only 6 child diagnoses; the DSM-IV has 41. Thus, the field of child psychopathology is relatively new.

Prevalence. Using DSM-III criteria, researchers in New Zealand found that approximately 25% of children aged 11-12 years met criteria for some diagnosis, which is similar to results from a sample of 15-year-olds. More than half were diagnosed with multiple disorders; the most common co-morbid disorders were attention-deficit in combination with either conduct disorder or oppositional defiant disorder. This finding is consistent with U.S. samples. Parents are most likely to seek help for conduct problems and hyperactivity. The Thinking About Gender Issues: Gender Differences Across Disorders box on page 454 addresses the issue of boys outnumbering girls in all disorders except anxieties and phobias during childhood, with girls displaying more problems during adolescence. These differences are explored in the context of boys' greater vulnerability of males to physical and psychological difficulties.

Oppositional Defiant and Conduct Disorders

Description. The criteria for oppositional defiant disorder (ODD) are presented on page 455; the disorder is characterized by significant defiant and negative child behavior, including frequent anger, temper tantrums, swearing, and defiance of adult rules. These symptoms are more apparent in the home and with children they know well, and usually appear before age 8. In serious cases, they may evolve into conduct disorder (CD), which is characterized by a repetitive and persistent pattern of conduct that violates the basic rights of others and major age-appropriate societal norms or rules (see page 456 for DSM-IV criteria). CD children may be verbally or physically aggressive, destructive of property, and cruel to animals. As children age, their aggression may include mugging, purse snatching, rape and murder. Violence is linked to conduct disorder. After age 18, behavior may include physical fights, reckless behavior, promiscuity, financial irresponsibility, and lack of guilt about their behavior; this will lead to a diagnosis of antisocial personality disorder. Many persons diagnosed with ODD or

CD demonstrate stable behavior problems into teen and adult years; a disproportionate number of adults with drug dependence report symptoms of CD and attentional problems during childhood. ODD is more common in boys: prevalence estimates range from 6-16% for males and 2-9% in females under age 18. CD individuals are often delinquent (persons under age 18 who have committed a legal offense). Most habitual offenders meet criteria for CD.

Causes. Genetic factors have been linked to aggressive behavior in twin studies via personality traits which may influence the display of aggression. Parents of CD children frequently display antisocial behavior (excessive drinking, criminal activity). Data suggest that impulsivity and low levels of anxiety, which may be stable predictors of adult aggression, may be linked to genetic and birth problems. Psychological determinants include learning, cognition and family factors which contribute to the development of CD and ODD. Aggressive behavior is likely to be rewarded by parents and peers. Nursery school children who behaved aggressively were more likely to receive positive consequences (i.e., get their way). Mother-child interactions have also been characterized by escalating punitive and negative interactions between mothers and their aggressive sons. Exposure to aggression through observing others (in real life or on TV) has been linked to aggressive behavior in children. Cognitive factors may facilitate aggression, as aggressive children may misperceive the intentions of others as hostile. Strong and frequent punishment by parents has also been associated with conduct problems and delinquent behavior. In addition, parents may explicitly encourage aggression outside the home, may be inconsistent and lax in their discipline, and may poorly monitor their children's behavior. Inept discipline is characterized by frequent and severe physical punishment, scolding and nagging in response to trivial problems, and failure to follow through on threats. Inept monitoring is characterized by the failure to provide adequate supervision and attention during child care. Patterson and Bank's model is presented on page 459: inconsistent punishment of coercive child behavior leads to occasional reinforcement of these behaviors; inept discipline and inept monitoring lead to antisocial behavior in children through an interactive process. Marital discord may be associated with child conduct problems because of modeling of hostility and aggression, aggression towards the child, or poor parent-child relationships. Social factors also are important, as children in lower SES groups have disproportionate rates of conduct problems and delinquent behavior. This relationship, however, may be due to large family size, poor parental discipline, and overcrowding. Stress plays a more direct and significant role in families headed by single mothers than in two-parent families.

Treatment. Patterson and colleagues have developed an effective treatment, parent training therapy. This involves teaching parents to praise desirable behavior (sharing & cooperating), ignore certain annoying or undesirable behaviors, and to punish other undesired behavior (swearing, talking back) through loss of privileges or isolation in the child's room for a fixed period. Coping strategies to deal with specific problem situations (i.e., homework) and the parents' own problems are also included. Because it is so difficult to change aggressive behavior in boys aged 9-12 years, there is an emphasis on early treatment and prevention. More positive outcome is associated with the absence of parental psychopathology and severe discord, frequent supportive contacts between mothers and their relatives and friends, and parental use of social learning concepts. Behavioral family systems therapy is used with aggressive behavior problems in children and adolescents, through increasing mutual reinforcement, communication, and negotiation in the family. This treatment has been shown to yield in a lower recidivism rate (rate of relapse or repeat offending) than no-treatment and alternative treatment. A home-style approach using house parents with adolescent delinquents is also effectively initially; however, gains are lost when the youths are returned to their homes. Problem-solving training (or cognitive skills training) focuses on the individual's cognitive processes, such as expectations, self-statements, taking the perspective of others, and problem-solving skills. If parents are included, a major focus is on improving the problem-solving process and emotional reactions of family members. Cognitive style, self-reports of behavior at home, communication, court referrals, and classroom behavior have shown improvement with this treatment. Severe aggression and delinquent behavior, remain difficult to change. Aggressive males who are accepted by their peers are less likely to change with treatment relative to those rejected by their peers. However, improved aggressive behavior in rejected boys is not likely to lead to increased peer acceptance. The use of medication with conduct problem children is controversial, as stimulants are usually ineffective.

Attention-Deficit/Hyperactivity Disorder (AD/HD)

The DSM-IV criteria are presented on page 463. AD/HD emerged as formal schooling became required for all children. The essential features of inattention, impulsiveness, and hyperactivity must have persisted for at least 6 months, and children are diagnosed as one of three subtypes: AD/HD; AD/HD, predominantly inattention type; or AD/HD, predominantly hyperactive-impulsive type. AD/HD is seen as a potentially lifelong problem; aggression is a better predictor of adult functioning than are hyperactivity or attention problems. Hyperactive children have a greater likelihood of having attention-deficit problems as adults, for developing antisocial personality disorder, and for drug abuse during adulthood.

Causes. A genetic predisposition is supported by the higher rate of AD/HD in parents and siblings of children with AD/HD, and by greater similarity in activity level among identical twins than in fraternal twins. Dietary influences, such as food dyes and additives (salicylates), were thought to cause hyperactivity in children. Controlled studies of the Feingold diet, however, failed to support this theory. Lead poisoning has been found to cause neurological problems and severe hyperactivity; this may occur through ingestion of chips of lead-based paint, and inhalation of lead fumes. Brain dysfunction was studied through EEGs and neurological exams; when these methods failed to yield significant findings, the term minimal brain dysfunction was used to describe very minor brain dysfunction that was thought to cause hyperactivity and motor coordination difficulties but which could not be detected directly. However, more recent research has suggested that brain dysfunction (such as decreased blood flow to the frontal lobes, abnormalities in the premotor and superior prefrontal cortex) may be linked to hyperactivity and attention problems. Psychological causes may influence the development of AD/HD, but are not primary causes of the disorder. Some of the same factors linked to conduct problems can influence AD/HD. More powerful incentives for appropriate behavior and at least some negative feedback for inappropriate behavior are necessary with hyperactive children. The primary symptoms of hyperactivity and inattention have not been linked to family or environmental factors; however, secondary symptoms of aggression and self-esteem in AD/HD children have been linked to short temper of the father, overly busy parents, poor parent-child relationship, urban residence, and low SES. Newborns at risk for brain dysfunction (premature birth, lack of oxygen) who had families with high emotional support, structure and organization displayed lower rates of behavior problems at age 10 compared to at-risk newborns from families with poor parental mental health, poor mother-child relationships and punitive child-rearing practices. Some of the parents' behavior, however, may be the result of the AD/HD children's effects on their parents; but even when AD/HD children become more attentive and compliant, parents do not increase rewarding or supportive comments. Thus, the influence of AD/HD children and parents on each other is unclear.

Treatment. Pharmacological treatment is most likely to involve psychostimulants, which increase certain brain functions that improve attention span and fine motor control. Ritalin and Cylert are the most common stimulants. Initially psychostimulant medication was thought to have a paradoxical effect because it was thought to stimulate or activate a center of the brain while producing a calming effect. However, children with no activity or attention problems respond in the same was as AD/HD children, with improved attention and fine motor skills. It is difficult to determine the exact effect of psychostimulant medication. Those with frontal abnormalities may show the greatest clinical improvement; other factors, such as type and severity of symptoms, developmental and intellectual factors, medical history, and family history of psychopathology may also affect treatment response. Other medications have also been used with AD/HD with some efficacy. Antidepressants are considered the second-line treatment, and may be most appropriate with AD/HD children displaying anxiety and/or depression. Antidepressants, however, are usually less effective than psychostimulants and have side effects. Medication in combination with some type of behavioral treatment is more effective than medication alone. Behavioral treatment has been successful in classroom settings. These typically involved praise for appropriate behavior (attending to and completing schoolwork), ignoring inappropriate behavior such as calling out answers, making classroom rules explicit and reviewing them daily, giving negative feedback privately, setting daily goals, providing daily feedback to parents, and requesting that parents reward children for meeting daily goals. Combined pharmacological and psychological treatment does lead to improvements. Treatment may also include tutoring, family therapy, and individual therapy for parents. Combined treatments appear to be most effective with those AD/HD children who display multiple symptoms (e.g., aggression and AD/HD). When conduct problems are significant, behavior therapy is often recommended; when attention problems and overactivity are primary, psychostimulant medication is recommended.

Anxiety Disorders

Description. Fears and worries are common among young children, and the number and type of fears change with age. Overanxious disorder (OD) is characterized by excessive worrying about new and future situations, such as being hurt, doing poorly on a test, or being criticized by others. OD children are unable to control their worrying, and may be irritable and have difficulty concentrating. OD occurs in families with high pressure to do well in school, and is more likely to occur in older children. Separation anxiety disorder is characterized by excessive anxiety concerning separation from the home or loved one. School phobia is characterized by a child's specific reluctance or refusal to go to school due to fear of separating from parents; this is a subclass of separation anxiety disorder. Longitudinal research with children demonstrates that childhood anxiety and fearfulness are likely to continue. Children with anxiety disorders are less likely to be brought for treatment, perhaps because they do not readily express their fears to parents, who may then be unaware of the nature and/or severity of their anxiety.

Causes. Family studies have shown that children of anxious parents are more likely to have anxiety symptoms than children of depressed parents. Parents with panic disorder are more likely to have children with anxiety problems than parents with generalized anxiety. Twin studies have provided convincing evidence of genetic factors; introversion and being anxious have high genetic components. Psychological determinants have long been thought to influence the development of anxiety in children. Watson's study of "Little Albert" demonstrated the role of classical conditioning. This view was modified to include preparedness, or the biological predisposition to react fearfully to certain stimuli and not others. Modeling or observing others has been supported as a contributing factor, as is reinforcement for fearful behavior (which may be accidental). Psychodynamic models emphasize dependency that is reinforced by parental attention (e.g., with school phobia).

Treatment. Mary Cover Jones' classic study demonstrated that exposure to peers who are unafraid can decrease fear in phobic children. Observing filmed models of children who gradually approach feared objects, use of self-statements (i.e., "I am brave") and reinforcement for brave behavior have been effective in reducing children's fears. Overanxious disorders are more difficult to treat than fears. Use of other children as "therapists," teaching perspective-taking skills, and social skills training (often with peer coaches, behavioral rehearsal, and coaching) may be helpful in reducing anxiety. However, children's popularity or peer acceptance may not change as a result of this treatment. Play therapy has been used with anxious and withdrawn children. The Thinking About Research: Does Play Therapy Work? box on page 474 examines this approach. Given the overlap between anxiety disorders and depression, a cognitive-behavioral intervention has been recommended. This includes: affective education in which children learn to understand and differentiate between feelings; behavioral procedures, such as relaxation training and exposure techniques; cognitive interventions to help children improve self-monitoring and self-control; social skills training to help children improve peer relationships; and parental involvement. School phobia is best treated in the early stages. Treatment involving close collaboration among the therapist, parents, and school personnel, prompt and strong pressure to return to school, and acceptance and support from teachers, has been effective. Adolescents who refuse to go to school, claim they are afraid of school, and come from families characterized by marital discord have not been successfully treated with psychological methods. Antidepressant medication has yielded inconsistent results, but may be helpful for some adolescents.

Enuresis

Enuresis is diagnosed for children of at least 5 years of age when bed-wetting or involuntary discharge of urine occurs more than once a week for at least 3 consecutive months. If the frequency is less, but the bed-wetting causes significant distress or impairment in functioning, the diagnosis may still be made. Approximately 85-90% of children are continent by age 5; by age 10, 95% are continent and by adulthood, 98% are continent. Enuresis is much more common among males: twice as many boys as girls wet their beds at age 5 (7% of boys, 3% of girls); about 1-2% of adult males are enuretic, while enuresis is virtually nonexistent for adult females. Children are more likely to be enuretic if they are of low SES and if a parent was also enuretic. Only about 15% of enuretics between the ages of 5 and 19 spontaneously stopped wetting the bed each year in one study which followed children over a 15-year period. Thus, most parents of school-aged enuretic children are advised to seek treatment. If parents mistakenly believe that their child is merely lazy, they may use shame or become angry at the child. Teasing and restricted ability to stay overnight with friends, relatives or go to camp may also be problems for enuretic children.

Causes. Parents may mistakenly believe that enuresis is caused by emotional problems or by extremely deep sleep that prevents children from detecting bladder pressure. Disease and infection account for only a small number of cases. Most bed-wetters fail to respond to cues from their bladders.

Treatment. The most effective method is the bell and pad method. This involves an alarm device that awakens a bed-wetter immediately upon urination so the child can get up and continue urination in the bathroom. The child may change the sheets, monitor progress on a daily chart, and may receive rewards for remaining dry. Most children (about 2/3) no longer wet the bed after 3 to 8 weeks of treatment. An all-night training program of intensive training is the dry bed training program. The child drinks large amounts of fluid before going to bed to increase the probability of urinating during the night, and a therapist is present. The child receives practice and positive reinforcement for getting out of bed to urinate, is reprimanded for accidents and must clean and remake the bed. In combination with the bell and pad method, approximately 80% of children are successful. Children attending mental health clinics because of significant behavioral and emotional problems are less successful and may require more lengthy treatment. Imipramine, an antidepressant, does reduce the frequency of bed-wetting; however, it is not a cure for enuresis.

Learning Disorders

Description. Learning disorders (LDs) are characterized by academic, language, speech and motor skills that are substantially lower than would be expected based on a child's intellectual capacity. These include reading disorder, mathematics disorder, and disorder of written expression. Reading disorder, also known as dyslexia, is characterized by impaired word-recognition skills and reading comprehension. Individuals tend to omit, add or distort works when reading, and read slowly and haltingly. Mathematics disorder is characterized by difficulty in understanding mathematical terms and operations and/or in recognizing numerical symbols and arithmetic signs. Inability to count, follow sequential steps, and learn multiplication tables are common. Disorder of written expression is evident by marked impairment in the development of expressive writing skills, which interferes significantly with the child's academic achievement or with daily activities that require expressive writing. Children with this disorder often produce writing that is poorly organized, grammatically incorrect, incorrectly punctuated, and with spelling errors. Less is known about this disorder, which often occurs in combination with reading disorder or mathematics disorder. Low self-esteem and difficulty getting along with others may accompany learning disorders. Approximately 40% drop out of school and problems at work may be present in adults with LD. Many children with LD also have conduct and oppositional disorders.

Causes. Some believe that neuropsychological problems will eventually be detected in LD persons. Others believe that LD represents the lower end of the distribution of abilities or is the result of developmental delays. There may be a genetic contribution to LD, perhaps involving chromosome 6. Underlying abnormalities in cognitive processing, genetic predisposition, perinatal injury, and severe neurological and general medical conditions have all be hypothesized to be causes of LD.

Treatment. Dietary changes, individual psychotherapy, family therapy, educational tutoring, large muscle training regimens to aid neurological development, and optometric training have all be used to treat LD. Schools are required to develop individualized educational programs to meet children's special needs, which may involve extensive training in specific skills. Private educational resource centers may provide tutoring or remedial services. Optometric training may aid visual tracking and focusing, and speech therapy may aid articulation difficulties.

Depression

Description. Childhood depression, which has only recently been recognized, is characterized by depressed mood, low self-esteem, fatigue, somatic complaints, suicidal thoughts, and a sense of hopelessness. Rates do not differ for boys and girls, although by late adolescence, depression occurs more frequently among girls than among boys. The Thinking About Controversial Issues: Teen Pregnancy and Abortion on page 479 explores the effects of pregnancy on teenage girls. While the DSM-IV does not provide separate diagnostic criteria for adults and children, depressed children are less likely to commit suicide, biological correlates are not identical for children and adults, and children do not generally show positive responses to antidepressant medication. In addition, depressed girls differ from depressed boys (see Table 14.2 on page 480).

Causes. Family factors have been studied, partly in an effort to explain the increased risk of depression among close relatives of individuals who are depressed. Children with depressed parents are more likely to be depressed and to have problems with substance abuse, social functioning and school functioning than children of nondepressed parents. While young children of depressed parents are unlikely to be depressed (only 1 in 100), children aged 15-20 years, especially girls, are much more likely to be depressed. However, the rate of depression in children of depressed parents is only 1% for boys and 4% for girls. Thus, other factors appear to be important. Children of depressed parents were more likely to have negative thoughts about themselves than were children of a parent with a medical condition. Criticism by family members also appears to be an important factor to study. Psychosocial stressors and genetic predispositions appear to increase the risk for childhood depression. Psychological factors, such as low self-worth, self-blame and self-criticism (perhaps resulting from parental criticism) may be linked to childhood depression.

Treatment. Psychological treatments focus on changing negative cognitive style, improving self-esteem, and building social skills. No particular psychological treatment has been found to be superior in the treatment of childhood depression. A combination of cognitive-behavioral treatment and family treatment may be most effective. Pharmacological treatment is based largely on research with depressed adults. Antidepressant drugs, however, do not appear to be effective with depressed children.

KEY IDEAS & OBJECTIVES FOR STUDENTS

After reading the chapter, you should be able to answer the following questions:

1. How is the development of the recognition and study of psychological disorders of children characterized?

2. What is the prevalence of childhood disorders? Which are most common? Are multiple disorders common?

3. How does the prevalence of various disorders differ for boys and girls?

4. What are the characteristics and symptoms of oppositional defiant disorder (ODD) and conduct disorder (CD)?

5. What evidence exists for the heritability of aggression and other characteristics which may influence the development of aggression?

6. What is the relationship between psychological and social factors and aggressive behavior in children?

7. What treatments are effective for ODD and CD and what do they emphasize?

8. What are the primary characteristics of young children with attention-deficit/hyperactivity disorder (AD/HD)?

9. What are the characteristics of AD/HD during childhood, adolescence, and young adulthood?

10. How does the coexistence of aggression and attentional problems affect prognosis?

11. What is the etiology of ADHD? What factors are related to aggressive problems in AD/HD children?

12. How are psychological and pharmacological therapies used in treating children with problems of attention and overactivity? Are they effective?

13. How does the prevalence of anxiety problems vary with gender?

14. How do genetic factors, conditioning, modeling, reinforcement, and complex cognitive learning affect the etiology of anxiety?

15. What psychological therapies are used to treat anxious children? Are they effective?

16. What factors are related to the development of enuresis?

17. What treatments are effective treating enuresis?

18. What are the characteristics and types of learning disorders (LD)?

19. What causes learning disorders?

20. What treatments are used for learning disorders? Do they lead to improvement?

21. What is the history of the study of childhood depression?

22. What are the risk factors for a child developing depression? How common is suicide among children?

23. What treatments are used for childhood depression? Is medication effective for children?

Using Case Studies in Abnormal Psychology by Meyer & Osborne:
Attention-Deficit Hyperactivity, Separation Anxiety, and Oppositional Defiant Disorders

Chapter 14 of the casebook presents several cases to illustrate disorders of childhood and adolescence. Developmental language disorder is portrayed in the case of Delano. Attention-Deficit Hyperactivity Disorder is illustrated in the case of Matt, and separation anxiety disorder associated with school refusal is covered in the case of Julie. Lastly, oppositional defiant disorder is addressed in the case of Phyllis. (Note: Autistic disorder is also covered in this chapter; however, this disorder is covered in chapter 15 of the text.)

Case Comparisons

Developmental Language Disorder: The Case of Delano. Delano was evaluated because of academic difficulties in first grade. Results indicated average intelligence, but specific deficits in receptive and expressive language, which adversely affected his reading ability. He, therefore, met criteria for Mixed Expressive-Receptive Language Disorder, and Reading Disorder. The characteristics of learning disorders are presented on page 477 of the text. Provide a summary of the specific characteristics of Del that support his diagnosis. Are any of the criteria questionable? Did Del display any characteristics of conduct problems? Support your answer with specific examples. What factors may have contributed to Del's learning disorder? Which theoretical models are linked to these factors? What treatment options were considered? Which were used?

Attention-Deficit Hyperactivity Disorder: The Case of Matt. The diagnostic criteria for AD/HD are presented on page 463 of the text. Provide a summary of the specific characteristics of Matt which support the diagnosis using each of the criteria. Which subtype of AD/HD did Matt exhibit? Are any of the criteria questionable? Did Matt meet the criteria for ODD or CD? Support your answers with specific examples. What factors may have led to the development of this problem? Which theoretical models are linked to these factors? Which treatments were considered? Which were used?

Separation Anxiety Disorder Associated With School Refusal: The Case of Julie. Julie, a second-grader with persistent refusal to attend school which resulted in court-ordered treatment, first exhibited difficulty attending school in first grade. The characteristics of separation anxiety disorder and school phobia are presented on page 471 of the text. Which characteristics did Julie (and her mother) display? Are any of the characteristics questionable? Support your answers with specific examples. What factors may have contributed to the development of this disorder for Julie? Which theoretical models are linked to these factors? What treatment options were considered? Which were used?

Oppositional Defiant Disorder: The Case of Phyllis. Phyllis is a teenager who displayed a consistent history of oppositional and defiant behavior. The characteristics of ODD are presented on page 455 of the text. Provide a summary of the specific characteristics of ODD displayed by Phyllis. Are any of the criteria questionable? Support your answer with specific examples. Treatment involved Adlerian and Gestalt techniques, followed by weekly group therapy with other adolescents. While these treatments are not covered explicitly in the text, students should be able to discuss treatment options discussed in the text and how they are (or are re not) consistent with the treatment Phyllis received.

Integrating Perspectives
A Biopsychosocial Model

The Case of Matt

Biological Factors

- Matt was always more "active" than other children from the start.
- Matt had greater difficulty than most children with respect to sustained concentration and attention.

Psychological Factors

- Psychological factors played less of a role in the development of the problem, but were critical for treatment. Matt's parents were asked to push Matt to slow his pace on difficult tasks and to make plans before beginning a task. His parents needed to be very consistent and systematic in these plans

Social Factors

- Our education system requires a certain that the individual be able to maintain a certain amount of attentiveness in order to benefit from the instruction.

Sample Multiple-Choice Questions

1. If you were a music teacher in New Zealand or the U.S. and you worked with 200 children, you would expect that about ________ of them would be diagnosed with some disorder and about ________ of these children with a diagnosis would have multiple disorders.
   a. 10 percent, 50 percent
   b. 15 percent, 10 percent
   c. 25 percent, 50 percent
   d. 40 percent, 10 percent

2. Randall is a 7-year-old child who has frequent temper tantrums and often blames his older brother for getting him in trouble for breaking family rules. He is able to follow rules at school fairly well, but argues with two boys from his class who live in his neighborhood. Randall's diagnosis is most likely ________.
   a. attention-deficit/hyperactivity disorder
   b. oppositional defiant disorder
   c. conduct disorder
   d. antisocial personality disorder

3. ________ discipline refers to frequent and severe physical punishment, such as grabbing, hitting, or beating with an object, as well as scolding and nagging when trivial problems occur.
   a. Atypical
   b. Enmeshed
   c. Disengaged
   d. Inept

4. Daniel's parents fight constantly, but remain married and living together. Gil's parents used to fight constantly, but since their divorce a year ago they have been able to resolve their differences and get along reasonably well. Based on research, which of the following statements is most likely to be TRUE?
   a. Daniel and Gil are both at risk of developing antisocial behavior.
   b. Gil is more likely than Daniel to develop antisocial behavior.
   c. Daniel is more likely than Gil to develop antisocial behavior.
   d. Neither Daniel nor Gil is at risk of developing antisocial behavior.

5. Research by Lochman and colleagues (1985) has shown that _______ were more likely to change aggressive behavior.
   a. boys who were accepted by their peers
   b. boys who were rejected by their peers
   c. girls who were rejected by their peers
   d. girls who were accepted by their peers

6. Which of the following factors does not appear to be a cause of attention-deficit/hyperactivity disorder, but may affect the maintenance of symptoms of AD/HD?
   a. salicylates and food additives
   b. lack of negative consequences for misbehavior
   c. minimal brain dysfunction
   d. genetic predisposition

7. Behavioral treatments of children with AD/HD may include all of the following EXCEPT ________.
   a. giving praise and small rewards for completing schoolwork and paying attention
   b. ignoring of inappropriate behavior
   c. setting daily goals and reviewing classroom rules
   d. eliminating negative feedback for inappropriate behavior

8. Katy is a two-year-old girl who does appears to have relatively normal levels and types of fears. She is most likely to be afraid of ________.
   a. the dark
   b. imaginary creatures
   c. noises
   d. death

9. In the 1970s, the ________ model was modified to include the notion that humans are biologically prepared to react fearfully to certain stimuli, such as snakes and spiders, but not to others, such as geometric shapes or wall sockets.
   a. modeling
   b. classical conditioning
   c. unconscious conflict
   d. familial transmission

10. The most successful treatment for enuresis is ________.
   a. the bell and pad method
   b. imipramine
   c. rewards for not wetting the bed
   d. play therapy

Answer Key

1. c
2. b
3. d
4. c
5. b
6. b
7. d
8. c
9. b
10. a

CHAPTER 15 MENTAL RETARDATION AND AUTISTIC DISORDER

Mental Retardation

A Historical Overview. Mental retardation was described by Hippocrates and attributed to brain damage before and during birth. In ancient times, mentally retarded infants were sometimes killed. In the Middle Ages, they were tolerated, viewed as in league with the devil, and/or subjected to barbaric treatment. At the end of the 18th century, Jean-Marc Gaspard Itard and Edouard Seguin initiated more humane institutional care for the mentally retarded. By the mid-1800s, however, institutions were characterized by custodial care rather than by efforts to rehabilitate. Sterilization of the mentally retarded was quite common. The discovery of the relationship between metabolism deficits and mental retardation led to a focus on prevention and treatment of mental retardation. Scientific research was directed towards identifying, preventing, and/or treating the biological causes of mental retardation. In the U.S., the Kennedy family strove to raise awareness and concern for the mentally retarded and their families, and this led to the foundation of the Special Olympics.

Diagnosis of Mental Retardation. The DSM-IV criteria are presented on page 487. These include: subaverage intellectual functioning (usually IQ below 70); deficits in adaptive functioning in at least two areas (communication, self-care, home living, social/interpersonal skills, use of community resources, self-direction, functional academic skills, work, leisure, health, and safety); and onset prior to age 18. Four levels of mental retardation are specified. Mild mental retardation (IQ between 50-55 and 70) encompasses 85% of persons with mental retardation. Most individuals in this group develop relatively normal social and communication skills between birth and starting school, exhibit few to no obvious signs of impairment until tested in school, and are likely to develop academic skills at the 6th grade level by late teen years. They usually function independently, although they may require special support in times of high stress. Moderate mental retardation (IQ between 35-40 and 50-55) includes 10% of mentally retarded persons. Individuals usually learn to speak as young children and are able to benefit from vocational training and learn self-care with supervision. They may acquire minimal academic skills (2nd grade level), and may experience poor peer relationships because they are unable to acquire social and interpersonal skills. During adulthood, they may work in unskilled or semiskilled jobs in sheltered settings. Severe mental retardation (IQ 20-25 to 35-40) accounts for 3-4% of mentally retarded persons, who are characterized by little to no speech (although they may sometimes learn to recite the alphabet, count, read a few words). They may acquire minimal self-care skills and perform simple tasks in closely supervised environments, but they cannot live independently. They may live in the community with close supervision. Profound mental retardation (IQ below 20-25) occurs in 1-2% of mentally retarded persons. These individuals usually have identifiable neurological conditions, which may also cause severe physical deficits. They have marked perceptual problems, which combine with their intellectual functioning to make it extremely difficult for them to learn. They require life-long care in highly structured environments. Amniocentesis involves withdrawing a small amount of amniotic fluid to diagnose hereditary conditions (e.g., chromosomal abnormalities) during pregnancy.

The Epidemiology of Mental Retardation. The worldwide prevalence of mental retardation is approximately 1%; 2.5 million individuals in the U.S. exhibit mental retardation. Financial and social costs are substantial. Prevalence varies across age groups. Fewer than 1% are identified in preschool populations, as only the most severe forms of mental retardation are evident prior to school. The highest prevalence occurs in school-aged (10-18 years) children, when intellectual and academic performance are emphasized and evaluated. Approximately 75% of mentally retarded persons are adolescents or younger. Prevalence then declines steadily across the life span; many mildly retarded persons disappear into society and most severely and profoundly retarded persons die by middle age. Sex differences exist as well; the ratio is 1.5 males to 1 female. SES and mental retardation are inversely related. Inferior quality of prenatal care, impaired ability of parents to provide academic stimulation, and a greater likelihood that poor children will be placed in classes for the mentally retarded all contribute to the greater prevalence among low SES persons.

The Nature and Causes of Mental Retardation. Many mentally retarded individuals display additional problems which impair their functioning (i.e., vision, speech and locomotion may be impaired). Neuropsychological deficits which prevent reading, writing, speaking or perceiving are common among those in severe and profound categories of retardation. Prenatal factors include maternal illness (diabetes and high blood pressure), chronic alcohol or drug abuse during pregnancy, medication taken during pregnancy, and incompatibility between the mother's and child's blood. Fetal alcohol syndrome is associated with retardation and physical abnormalities. Viral infections during pregnancy, such as rubella, can cause both mental and physical impairment; although syphilis is no longer a major cause of mental retardation in the U.S., it can cause mental retardation.

Chromosomal mutations occurring prior to conception are more common among older mothers and fathers (e.g., over 40 years) and usually are found on autosomal chromosomes or sex chromosomes. Down syndrome usually causes moderate and severe mental retardation and usually produces distinct physical characteristics. Children with this disorder have small, rounded skulls with flattened, moon-shaped faces; openings for their eyes are narrow and have a downward and inward slope; their noses are short, their tongues are often large and may protrude from their mouths; their cheeks are rosy; and their hair may be coarse, wiry and sparse. They are usually small for their age. Mothers over the age of 32 have at least a seven times greater risk of having a child with Down syndrome. There are at least three different chromosomal abnormalities responsible for Down syndrome: trisomy 21 is the most common and is characterized by a third chromosome number 21, resulting in a total of 47 (rather than 46) total chromosomes. Approximately 1 in every 700 live births result in Down syndrome, but only 10% of these individuals live in institutions. Fewer than half have IQs greater than 50. They are cooperative, friendly, happy and easily managed during childhood. Emotional and behavioral disorders are more likely to develop during adolescence, including antisocial behavior, drug abuse, and sexual promiscuity; institutionalization is increasingly common during young adulthood.

Genetic defects account for about 5% of mental retardation. Alkaptonuria involves a disorder of amino acid formation. Phenylketonuria (PKU) is the most intensively studied, and involves the inability to convert phenylalanine into tyrosine; phenylalanine levels increase, which produce decreases in serotonin, epinephrine, and norepinephrine. The prevalence of PKU is 1 in every 10,000 to 20,000 persons in the U.S. Individuals are of small stature, with especially small heads; they tend to be hyperactive, to display temper tantrums and bizarre movements of the body and upper extremities, and are unlikely to develop verbal or nonverbal communication. Most become severely or profoundly retarded and seizures are likely. A screening test administered to newborns is effective in identifying potential PKU. A low phenylalanine diet can avoid most of the intellectual, behavioral, and physical problems. However, since phenylalanine is necessary for normal muscle growth and development, normal diet is resumed around age 6 when brain development is complete.

Postnatal factors involve accidents resulting from head injuries from automobile accidents and falls which cause brain damage that results in seizures and mental retardation. Prolonged oxygen deprivation (e.g., near drowning) and lead poisoning also cause mental retardation. Meningitis is an infection of the membrane covering the brain and encephalitis is an infection of the brain itself. Both can cause mental retardation.

Environmental factors may be important in the higher prevalence of mental retardation found among low SES individuals. Approximately 10-30% of low SES individuals meet the criteria for at least mild mental retardation. Familial mental retardation occurs when children born to mentally retarded parents are more likely to be mentally retarded. Level of retardation is usually mild and there is no evidence of CNS damage. In addition to the mental retardation, these parents are likely to pass on other problems, such as alcohol and drug abuse/dependence, juvenile and adult crime, promiscuity and teen pregnancy, and early school dropout.

Mental Retardation and Mental Illness. Mental disorders are more prevalent among the mentally retarded. These individuals may be more likely to come to the attention of mental health professionals who are then able to identify co-morbid mental disorders. Deficits in adaptive functioning from mental retardation may also be symptoms of other disorders, and behavioral and social limitations experienced may cause psychopathology. Most professionals, however, have not been trained to treat mental illness in mentally retarded individuals, and opportunities for treatment may be limited.

Prevention of Mental Retardation and Care for People Who Are Mentally Retarded. Prevention efforts include education about the nature and causes of mental retardation. Genetic counseling prior to and during pregnancy, nutrition and health practices during pregnancy, and modifying or eliminating environmental causes of brain damage may reduce the prevalence of mental retardation. Care at home and in public schools is another important area. Approximately 900,000 retarded children attend public school in the U.S., while only 110,000 children and adults live in institutions. Special education teachers and classes for the mentally retarded may facilitate learning, and programs to deal with associated behavioral and emotional problems are important. Emotional and intellectual development is usually better in a home environment than in an institution. However, children who are physically aggressive or delinquent may require institutionalization. Most treatment involves behavior therapy or cognitive-behavior therapy methods. This may include: identification of negative self-statements about intellectual, social and vocational abilities; adoption of more constructive and positive self-statements; and incorporation of more adaptive interpersonal and cognitive behavior. Research supports the efficacy of CBT.

Legislation has supported the rights of the mentally retarded (e.g., the 1985 Cleburne decision) and the need for appropriate community-based services. Public Law 94-142, the Education for All Handicapped Children, guaranteed the right to a free and appropriate education, an individualized educational program to be reevaluated annually, education in the least restrictive environment, and due process. Mainstreaming of mentally retarded children increased significantly as a result of this law. PL 99-457 extended these rights to children 3-5 years of age; this supported early intervention efforts, recognized the importance of the family, and eliminated categorizing labels because of their stigmatizing effect. PL 94-142 was updated in 1990 and renamed the Individuals with Disabilities Education Act; children with autism and traumatic brain injury were specifically included.

Care in institutions is still important for those individuals who cannot function in the home and school. Many facilities are publicly supported as private institutions are very expensive. Despite improvements in quality of public institutions, many are still overcrowded and underfunded. The use of major tranquilizers to sedate patients has decreased significantly. More transitional and community-based programs have also become available recently. The emphasis on community-based programs and deinstitutionalization of the mentally retarded, however, has been criticized because some individuals may not be able to function outside the institution. The Thinking About Controversial Issues box on page 499 explores this issue further by summarizing the conflict between those who wish to close an institution and place residents in community care and parents who feel their children need the level of structure and care provided in the institution.

Behavioral treatment of self-injury has been used with those who may repeatedly bang their heads with their hands, slap their faces, pick at their skin, pull their ears, or poke their eyes. Untreated, this may result in serious injury. Treatment includes: withholding social interaction with important persons in the retarded individual's environment as punishment; providing an enriched environment which acts as a distracter for self-injury; eliminating sensory feedback from self-injury by having the individual wear heavy clothing, thereby reducing the reinforcement value; punishing attempts at self-injury; and communication training. Each component has been demonstrated to be somewhat effective in reducing self-injury; however, none has been universally successful. Punishment is very controversial.

Behavior modification has been used in the form of token economies and other procedures to manage the behavior of patients. Tangible reinforcers are used for desired behaviors, while inappropriate behaviors are ignored or punished. Nondisabled peers have been trained to systematically reinforce appropriate behavior, and ignore or punish inappropriate behavior; retarded individuals are more responsive to nondisabled peers than to ward staff.

Autistic Disorder

The Nature of Autistic Disorder. Formerly called infantile autism, this disorder is characterized by marked impairment in social responsiveness, profound communications deficits, and stereotyped or bizarre habits and movements. The DSM-IV criteria for the disorder are presented on page 501. These include 3 major criteria. The first is qualitative impairment in social interaction evident by two of the following: marked impairment in use of multiple non-verbal behaviors such as eye-to-eye gaze, facial expression, body postures, and gestures to regulate social interaction; failure to develop peer relationships appropriate to developmental level; lack of spontaneous seeking to share enjoyment, interests, or achievements with other people (lack of showing, bringing, or pointing out objects of interest); and lack of social or emotional reciprocity. The second criteria is qualitative impairments in communication as manifested by at least one of the following: delay in, or total lack of, the development of spoken language (not accompanied by an attempt to compensate through alternative modes of communication such as gesture or mime); in individuals with adequate speech, marked impairment in the ability to initiate, or sustain a conversation with others; stereotyped and repetitive use of language or idiosyncratic language; and lack of varied, spontaneous make-believe imitative play appropriate to developmental level. The third involves restricted repetitive and stereotyped patterns of behavior, interests, and activities, as manifested by at least one of the following: encompassing preoccupation with one or more stereotyped and restricted patterns of interest that is abnormal either in intensity or focus; apparently inflexible adherence to specific, nonfunctional routines or rituals; stereotyped and repetitive motor mannerisms (hand or finger flapping or twisting, complex whole body movements); and persistent preoccupation with parts of objects. Symptoms occur prior to 30 months of age and the symptoms that are most troubling to parents are the social unresponsiveness. Approximately 50% remain mute; those with speech may display echolalia (mimicking others' speech), or pronoun reversal. By the time a child is 3 or 4 years old, parents are aware that the child has a problem, although they may believe that the problem is an emotional disturbance.

The Course of Autistic Disorder. Kanner first described autistic disorder in 1943. Prevalence is 2-5 children in 10,000, thus, it is a rare disorder. Most diagnosed between 1940-1970s did not receive highly specialized education or treatment. Studies of longterm outcome are based on these individuals. One study found that 42% were institutionalized, the majority were educationally impaired, 10-15% were of borderline intelligence, and 1-2% recovered. Other studies have also found that few are able to function independently in adulthood. Verbal skill is a better predictor of later functioning than general intelligence. Those with language show fewer symptoms of autism and may be able to complete high school or college, live at home or in a group setting, and maintain employment. A rare number may be an autistic savant, or a person who suffers from the full autistic disorder syndrome but also has some singular talent that usually emerges very quickly at an early age.

Causes of Autistic Disorder. There is no single cause of autistic disorder, but it does not appear to be caused by environmental factors; it is likely that one or more genetic/biological factors cause the disorder. Rutter's twin study supports a genetic transmission of autism and severe cognitive impairment. Siblings of autistic individuals are at significantly greater risk for the disorder than those without an autistic sibling. Autism probably results from a genetic predisposition to develop language and cognitive disorders, one of which is autism. Although many believe that several forms of brain dysfunction underlie autistic disorder, none has been confirmed to date. The inability to imitate significantly impairs language development and adversely affects social interactions. Endocrinal and chromosomal abnormalities have been found in some individuals, but not consistently. Psychological factors once were thought to cause autism, but few accept this view today. Kanner thought that parents who were detached and emotionally cold caused autism. Bruno Bettelheim suggested that autistic children be removed from their parents because they were unconsciously hostile, cold and rejecting as parents. Psychodynamic therapy is rarely provided today for autistic children and their families. Ferster, a behavioral psychologist, suggested that children unable to obtain attention and rewards for appropriate social behavior from their parents developed autism; this is not supported by research. More recent theories focus on the child's inability to comprehend complex social and interpersonal interactions because of a neurological defect in information processing. This view is consistent with the finding that autistic individuals have difficulty attending to a stimulus in the presence of other distracting stimuli.

Treatment of Autistic Disorder. Psychological methods are the primary means of treatment. Behavior therapy is effective in teaching language, social, and self-help skills. Teaching skills can take months and requires exceptional patience and perseverance. Children may first need to be taught to respond to simple requests, to attend, and to imitate. Ivar Lovaas has developed an intensive early intervention program for autistic children between the ages of 2 and 4 years, which requires 40+ hours per week of treatment. Although this program was effective in teaching language and self-help skills, children regressed once the intensive treatment was discontinued. About half the children were able to attend regular or special education classes in public schools, and 47% had normal range IQs. Only 2% of children in the control sample were at this same level. While intensive early intervention is costly, the costs of life-long institutionalization are much higher (e.g., up to $2 million). Others question the costs to the family, such as neglect by parents of other children in the home. Successful treatment requires basic teaching principles that imitate a child's behavior, uses parents as active teaching resources, works one-on-one with the child, makes aspects of the program home-based, and embraces a positive attitude as a meaningful component of the healing process. Punishment techniques used with autistic individuals are very controversial. The Thinking About Controversial Issues box on page 508 addresses this issue.

Pharmacological methods have included different medications, none of which has been effective for the majority of children. Psychostimulant medication to increase attention span has been used to reduce attention-deficit hyperactivity problems; however, other symptoms may worsen with this medication. Haloperidol, an antipsychotic medication, has been used to decrease severe aggressive and self-injurious behavior. Many negative side effects and risk of seizures, and the failure to ameliorate social withdrawal, abnormal interpersonal relationships, and cognitive deficits limit the utility of this drug. Anticonvulsant medication may be used, as 25% have a seizure disorder. Because 30-40% of autistic children may have elevated serotonin, fenfluramine, an antipsychotic medication, has been used; about 1/3 of individuals on this drug showed "strong improvement" and 1/2 showed some improvement in responsivity to the environment, stereotyped habit patterns and increased attention and eye contact. IQ score increases (verbal and performance) were observed. However, other studies have failed to find improvement with this drug, although serotonin levels have been shown to decrease with medication.

Curing Autistic Disorder. A cure for the disorder would entail the following: all unusual behaviors gone, the individual would have speech, would initiate social contact, and would interact with others. In the case of Noah presented in this chapter, a father of an autistic child describes his anger and frustration at those who believe that there is a cure for autistic disorder. Raun Kaufman's son's dramatic improvement represents one of these cases of an apparent cure for autism. Despite these case reports, it is unclear how many children will make such dramatic improvements, and it remains unclear which children will have such success.

KEY IDEAS AND OBJECTIVES FOR STUDENTS

After reading the chapter, you should be able to answer each of the following questions:

1. What is the prevalence of mental retardation?

2. What is the history of the study and care of the mentally retarded?

3. What are the symptoms and characteristics of persons diagnosed with mental retardation?

4. What are the characteristics of the four degrees of severity of mental retardation specified by the DSM-IV?

5. How does the prevalence of mental retardation vary with age and SES?

6. What causes mental retardation?

7. How often does mental illness occur in the mentally retarded?

8. Are prevention efforts successful in reducing the rate of mental retardation?

9. How are prevention activities conducted to reduce the incidence of mental retardation?

10. How have advances in institutional and home care affected the ability of mentally retarded individuals to live?

11. What are the characteristics of self-injury in the mentally retarded and how is it treated?

12. What are the characteristics and symptoms of children with autistic disorder?

13. What is the prevalence of autistic disorder? What is the relationship with mental retardation and what is the best predictor of later functioning?

14. What are the characteristics of an autistic savant?

15. What causes autistic disorder? Is it genetically transmitted?

16. Are psychological factors linked to autistic disorder?

17. What are the primary means of autistic children?

18. How is behavior therapy used with children with autism, and is it effective?

19. How difficult is teaching simple skills to autistic children?

20. How effective are pharmacological methods for treating autistic disorder?

21. Can autistics disorder be cured?

Mental Retardation and Autistic Disorder in the Movies

1. Rain Man (1980, MGM/UA, 134 min). The character in this film (portrayed by Dustin Hoffman) is an adult male with autistic disorder. The character also displays autistic savant abilities (e.g., exceptional memory, ability to count and estimate mathematical probabilities). Many of the characteristics of autistic disorder are demonstrated in this film. Impaired social interactions are exhibited through poor eye contact, flat affect, lack of spontaneous sharing with others, lack of peer relationships, and lack of emotional reciprocity. Language and communication deficits are also portrayed: although Raymond has speech, he demonstrates delayed echolalia, little initiation of speech, and repetitive use of language. Stereotyped behavior is evident in restricted patterns of interest (recording events in a notebook), inflexibility (watching Judge Wapner on People's Court, arrangement of his bed), and repetitive motor movements (body rocking and hand-flapping). Occasional self-injurious behavior is also evident. While Raymond is relatively high functioning, it is evident that he is not capable of independent living. Students can identify many of the symptoms and behaviors associated with this disorder. The film may also serve to prompt a consideration of long-term outcome and the difficulties in finding an appropriate placement for autistic adults.

Questions after watching the movie:

1. Given the text's description of the symptoms and associated behaviors of an individual with autistic disorder, how well did the movie do in presenting an accurate portrayal of this disorder? What "errors" (including errors of omission and commission) were made?

2. Although the film did not deal with the etiology of the disorder, what would contemporary theories suggest about the etiology?

3. Are there any other disorders displayed by Raymond? What is his intellectual functioning?

4. Although the film did not address treatment (other than living in an institution), what treatments would you recommend for this individual?

5. If you were to be a consultant on a "remake" of this film, what advice would you give the director to help make the symptoms, etiology, and treatment more contemporary?

2. Dominick and Eugene (1988, Orion Home Video, 111 min). This film portrays the relationship between two brothers, one of whom is mentally retarded. The older, normal brother (played by Ray Liotta) must come to terms with the special needs of his brother (played by Tom Hulce), who is mildly mentally retarded. The film does illustrates nicely the level of functioning of many adults with mild mental retardation, and their abilities to function in the community with support. The limitations of the mentally retarded individual and the need for special support in order to function are portrayed and could help students appreciate the level of functioning of the majority of the mentally retarded individuals in the U.S. The film could also serve as a prompt for considering how families choose the appropriate care for the

mentally retarded individual, and the extent to which the mentally retarded adult should participate in that choice.

Questions after watching the movie:

1. Given the text's description of the symptoms and associate behavior of individuals with mild mental retardation, how well did the movie doe in presenting an accurate portrayal of this disorder? What "errors" (including errors or omission and commission) were made?

2. Although the film did not deal with the etiology of the disorder, what would contemporary theories suggest about the etiology?

3. Are there any other disorders displayed?

4. How well did the film present treatments and alternative living arrangements? What treatments and living conditions would you recommend for this individual?

5. If you were to be a consultant on a "remake" of this film, what advice would you give the director to help make the symptoms, etiology, and treatment more contemporary?

Using Case Studies in Abnormal Psychology by Meyer & Osborne:
Autism

Chapter 14 of the casebook covers disorders of childhood and adolescence. The case of Audrey illustrates autistic disorder. The difficulty in distinguishing between autistic disorder and mental retardation is addressed first, and a comparison between children with autistic disorder alone, mental retardation alone, and both autistic disorder and mental retardation is discussed. The case of Audrey illustrates a child with both autistic disorder and mental retardation, which occurs most frequently with autistic disorder.

Autistic Disorder: The Case of Audrey. Audrey exhibited signs of difficulty from a very early age, which gradually led to increasing concern by her parents that their daughter was not normal. Although they raised these concerns with their pediatrician, Audrey was not evaluated fully and formally diagnosed until she was several years old. The characteristics of mental retardation are presented in the text on page 487 and the characteristics of autistic disorder are presented on page 501. Provide a summary of the specific characteristics of Audrey that support her diagnosis of autism. Are any of the criteria questionable? Does Audrey exhibit any of the characteristics of mental retardation? Be sure to provide specific examples to support your answers. What factors may have contributed to the development of this disorder for Audrey? What treatment options were considered? Which were used? Given the level of Audrey's functioning at age 5, can you estimate what her ultimate functioning might be?

Integrating Perspectives
A Biopsychosocial Model

The Case of Audrey

Biological Factors

- Audrey was born full-term, but from the start she seemed less responsive to her mother. In particular she did not respond to being held. Rather than "molding" herself when cradled in her mother's arms, she was stiff and rigid.
- Much of Audrey's physical development seemed to advance at a somewhat accelerated pace. However, she did not vocalize as consistently as most children. It was difficult to get her to engage in make-believe baby talk.

Psychological Factors

- Change in the environment seemed to frighten her. Audrey did not make friends. She was content to play alone for hours at a time.

Social Factors

- Audrey seemed unresponsive to any social factors.

Sample Multiple-Choice Questions

1. Mental retardation affects approximately _____ percent of the population in the United States.
   a. 1
   b. 2
   c. 5
   d. 10

2. Joanna is in the second grade. She is unable to count, do basic addition, recite the alphabet, tell time, or identify basic colors. According to her teachers and a number of standardized tests, Joanna appears to be delayed in __________ development when compared to her same-aged peers.
   a. intellectual
   b. adaptive
   c. communicative
   d. interpersonal

3. Stacie is unaware that she is pregnant with her first child. Stacie is a college student who likes to party at least 3 or 4 days a week. When she parties, she typically drinks 5 or more alcoholic beverages within a three-hour period. Lately, Stacie has been vomiting more than average in the mornings, which she attributes to drinking more than she usually does. Stacie's baby has an increased risk of developing ___________.
   a. rubella
   b. autism
   c. fetal alcohol syndrome
   d. chromosomal mutations

4. Mentally retarded persons are at ________ risk for developing mental illness, compared to nonretarded persons.
   a. lower
   b. equal
   c. greater
   d. unknown; there is not sufficient information to determine their risk

5. Approximately ________ percent of mentally retarded persons live in institutions.
   a. 10
   b. 25
   c. 30
   d. 50

6. Marcie is institutionalized for mental retardation. She frequently bangs her head with her hands, slaps her own face, and picks at her skin. These behaviors, referred to as ______________ behaviors, may cause permanent damage.
   a. fatalistic
   b. self-injurious
   c. severe
   d. disease-oriented

7. Approximately _______ percent of autistic individuals remain speechless throughout their lives.
   a. 10
   b. 25
   c. 33
   d. 50

8. Marcie has autistic disorder. Her parents have asked how she will continue to develop. Her therapist explains that research has found _______________ to be the best predictor of later functioning for children with autism.
   a. verbal ability
   b. interpersonal support
   c. motor ability
   d. cognitive ability

9. A(n) _________________ person is someone who suffers from the full autistic disorder syndrome, but also has some singular talent that usually emerges at an early age.
   a. learning disabled
   b. mentally retarded
   c. borderline autistic
   d. autistic savant

10. Zoe has been diagnosed with autistic disorder. What will be the primary means of treatment for Zoe?
   a. psychological interventions
   b. pharmacological treatment
   c. radiation treatment
   d. institutionalization

Answer Key

1. a
2. a
3. c
4. c
5. a
6. b
7. d
8. a
9. d
10. a

CHAPTER 16 COGNITIVE DISORDERS

Normal Aging, Healthy Aging

Psychologists such as Powell and Whitla have explored differences in how cognition is impacted by normal aging versus Alzheimer's disease. This disease is a brain disorder of pathological aging characterized by a profound, progressive loss in cognitive ability.

People today live longer and enjoy better health--by the year 2000, more than 1 in 10 Americans will be older than 65 (compared to 1 in 25 in 1900). The population of persons 65 and older is growing at a rate of 21% and at 37% for those over age 75 as compared to 12.5% for the rest of the population. Between 2010 and 2030, the numbers of Americans over age 65 will increase by 73% while the rest of the population will decrease by 3%. Society is aging rapidly because: 1) people are having fewer children, 2) society's growing concern for healthier lifestyles, and 3) advances in medicine (e.g., new drugs to treat chronic conditions that cause premature deaths. Seventy- and eighty-year-olds live active, productive lives and are fully interested in learning, producing, and remaining fully involved in society. A number of organizations, such as the American Psychological Association, have recently joined together to create a program to research key issues that society will confront as America ages (e.g., health, the very old, work, and psychological well-being). The MacArthur Foundation in one group in the US that has begun to research and identify the genetic, physiological, psychological, and social factors contributing to successful aging, or the process in which elderly deal successfully deal with issues common in old age (e.g., loss of lifelong partner, chronic illness). In the late 1980s, Medicare legislation increased funding for home health services, acute care, and long-term coverage allowing many elderly to remain in their homes and maintain their independence. In 1995, the future of Medicare seems to be in jeopardy. Federal and state governments have also begun confronting ageism, which involves prejudicial attitudes, discriminatory practices, and institutional policies directed against certain people solely because of their age. Women are especially susceptible to the problems posed by ageism (e.g., more likely than men to fall into poverty in their old age and less likely to be aware of available social services and financial aids). Powell and Whitla proposed 4 measures of normal cognitive aging or the normal impact of the aging process on thinking, problem solving, and remembering. These measures are age-group normative, probably not impaired, reference-group normative, and reference-group plus.

Cognitive Disorders

The fundamental disturbance in the cognitive disorders "is a clinically significant deficit in cognition or memory that represents a significant change from a previous level of functioning." A distinct collection of symptoms that often occur together is called a syndrome. One or more cognitive syndromes comprise every cognitive disorder. Delirium and dementia are the most common and most significant cognitive syndromes. Delirium is caused by brain injury and accompanies metabolic or toxic brain disturbances, including infections that cause high fevers; reduction in oxygen supply to the brain; and alcohol or other drug intoxication. Persons with delirium often don't know what time it is or where they are, can't pay attention for more than a few minutes, may experience hallucinations, and are also typically restless and agitated, constantly moving without purpose. Dementia results from strokes (which deprive parts of the brain of oxygen for long enough periods to cause their death); certain serious infections, like syphilis and human immunodeficiency virus (HIV); and brain tumors, brain injury, and chronic, progressive brain diseases. Persons with dementia experience a global deterioration in their intellectual, emotional, and cognitive abilities. They have difficulties performing tasks that require them to remember, learn, or use facts. Also typical of dementia are changes in personality, emotional balance, and mood however, memory loss is usually the initial sign of the syndrome. Paranoid delusions are common as dementia progresses. The primary impairments in amnestic disorder are in remembering and perceiving. Very remote events are typically remembered better than those that took place a few days, weeks, or months ago. Amnestic disorder can be caused by head trauma, alcohol abuse, malnutrition, brain surgery, oxygen deprivation, stroke, or brain infection. Research has localized the brain damage responsible for most amnestic disorders to the medial portions of the diencephalon.

Acute cognitive disorders are mild disorders, lasting only a few minutes or hours with complete recovery occurring in almost all cases, with only slight or nonexistent permanent effects (e.g., delirium that young children with high fevers sometimes experience). Chronic cognitive disorders, like Alzheimer's disease, are typically irreversible, last a long time, and generally have serious behavioral consequences.

Historical Overview

Cognitive disorders that result from pathological aging, chronic substance abuse, and certain physical diseases have been recognized throughout most of history. Yet, the precise nature of the changes in brain structure and function that cause them has only recently been investigated. It was only in the 1800s that Emil Kraeplin concluded that the brain was centrally involved in the marked changes produced by these causes. The first focused attempt to understand the brain and its role in behavior is generally traced to the early nineteenth century to German phrenologists Gall and Spurzheim. Phrenologists were quasi-scientists who studied the formation of the skull in the belief that it revealed a person's mental facilities and character. These researchers mapped protuberances on the head.

Efforts to investigate brain structure and localize brain function advanced significantly in the mid-nineteenth century when French surgeon Paul Broca studied posthumously the brains of two stroke patients whose ability to speak had been affected. Broca discovered that the posterior third of the inferior frontal convolution in each brain had been severely damaged by the stroke. This led him to conclude that speech is localized in this area of the brain, which has since been called Broca's area. A disorder called Broca's aphasia, is a disturbance in the comprehension and formulation of language caused by a dysfunction in Broca's area and neighboring brain regions. A few years after Broca's discovery, German physiologists Fritsch and Hitzig reported that when they electrically stimulated specific regions of a dog's cortex, specific voluntary muscles immediately contracted, confirming that specific brain regions control specific body movements (electrical stimulation method). French neurologist Jean Charcot exerted his greatest influence during the late-nineteenth century who systematically described the complex interplay of neurological and psychiatric symptoms in delirium, dementia, and other cognitive syndromes. Another Charcot pupil was George Gilles de la Tourette who later discovered Tourette's syndrome, a rare neurological syndrome in children. The study of the relationships between the brain and behavior has yielded tow paradoxical findings: 1) specific regions of the brain have been found to exert control over various bodily functions and 2) it is impossible to precisely identify the areas of the brain responsible for many bodily functions.

The Nature and Causes of Cognitive Disorders

Severe disruptions in a person's memory and thinking can result from minor changes in the brain. Likewise, striking alterations in the structure and function of the brain can sometimes produce surprisingly small behavioral changes. The form a person's brain disorder takes is based on a number of factors which are limited by the nature and extent of the brain damage: prior learning history, education, the emotional consequences of the brain injury, chronological and psychological maturity, and the intellectual competence of the person. Many cognitive disorders are life threatening; for example, death generally comes to patients with Alzheimer's disease within a decade of the initial appearance of its symptoms. There is also a greatly increased risk of depression and other mood disorders experienced by older people with cognitive disorders; about 30% of patients with Alzheimer's disease meet the DSM-IV diagnostic criteria for major depressive disorder. Depression and other emotional disorders may occur due to cognitive disorders seriously impairing quality of life in the final years. In addition, some cognitive disorders directly affect the brain areas that control people's experience and expression of mood. Many of the psychological consequences of the cognitive disorders diminish when the people who have them receive adequate social support from family and friends.

Assessment of Cognitive Disorders

Neuropsychological Procedures. In the 1930s and 1940s, a growing number of clinical psychologists became interested in assessing the intellectual and emotional consequences of brain damage, thus creating the subfield of clinical neuropsychology. Ward Halstead established the first human neuropsychology laboratory--the Halstead-Reitan Neuropsychological Battery. With his student, Ralph Reitan, he developed a neuropsychological test battery which remains the most widely used measure of cognitive functioning. Aleksander Luria, whose major work was done during the early part of the twentieth century, developed a detailed theory of cortical functioning on which the Luria-Nebraska Neuropsychological Battery was developed. This validity of this instrument continues to be debated.

Neuroimaging Techniques. The X-ray, discovered in the late 1800s by Roentgen, was the first technology created to allow us to look inside the living body. The use of contrast materials like air have extended the X-ray's usefulness for brain scientists. Pneumoencephalogram is a diagnostic procedure that employs air as an X-ray contrast medium to demonstrate brain contours. Because the procedure introduces a foreign substance into the body, however, it runs a modest risk of inducing infection or damage. Computerized axial tomography (CAT, CAT scan) revolutionized the clinical investigation of brain diseases because it provides detailed images of the living brain's gross cerebral structure. One of the first achievements of the CAT was to confirm long-held suspicion that the lateral and third ventricle spaces and some of the cortical surface markings of the brains of people with Alzheimer's disease were enlarged, whereas the brain tissue surrounding the ventricles was substantially reduced. Magnetic resonance imaging (MRI) provides extraordinarily clear reconstruction of the brain that does not require the use of ionizing radiation. The positron emission tomography (PET, PET scan) provides direct access to information on brain function. When used in conjunction with a CAT or MRI, a PET scan can help to localize a structural abnormality and then test for the functional consequences of the abnormality.

Cognitive Disorders Due To Pathological Aging

Dementia of the Alzheimer's Type has become a major public health problem in the United States and other developed countries. It is an age-related disorder characterized by profound, progressive losses in cognitive ability and marked changes in behavior and personality. It is the most common cause of cognitive disorder in the elderly, rates of Alzheimer's disease approximately double every 5 years beyond the ages of 65-70, and the prevalence of Alzheimer's disease in the U.S. population has been estimated at about 10% in persons over 65 and 45% in persons over 85.

Nature of the Dementia of the Alzheimer's Type. Dementia is an important feature of this disease. Significantly impaired short- and long-term memory is a conspicuous early symptom of dementia; it is commonly accompanied by disturbances in the ability to exercise sound judgment, think abstractly, and plan ahead. Other common features are aphasia (problems in understanding and using words, even familiar ones), apraxia (difficulties in moving parts of the body), and agnosia (impairments in the ability to recognize or identify familiar objects. A recent study reports that Alzheimer's patients who developed aphasia or apraxia deteriorated more rapidly than those without either symptom. Pronounced changes in behavior and personality generally develop slowly and the duration of dementia is typically years. Since problems of forgetfulness affect virtually everyone over the age of 50 or 60, an innovative test has been developed to distinguish between normal and pathological aging.

Alzheimer's disease is not simply accelerated aging; the effects of the disease on the brain and behavior of people who get it differ markedly from those of normal aging. Table 16.2 summarizes some of the ways in which clinicians distinguish between the effects on memory of normal (benign) and pathological (malignant) aging. Many people with Alzheimer's underestimate or deny their deficits for as long as they can; many more react with depression, anger, and frustration. The risk of depression is higher among Alzheimer's patients (30%). Because many of the symptoms of major depression mimic those of early dementia, differentiating depression from the early stages of dementia in the elderly is sometimes difficult. Individuals who are older and severely depressed may demonstrate depressive pseudodementia, a mood disorder in which the symptoms resemble those of dementia, but the condition is not a cognitive disorder. Treating these two conditions effectively requires greatly different approaches.

Causes of Dementia of the Alzheimer's Type. The brain of individual's with Alzheimer's disease invariably shows two significant features: 1) a generalized atrophy of the brain and, 2) the presence of foreign, nonfunctional cells (called neurofibrillary tangles, senile plaques, and granulovascular bodies). Sometimes these nonfunctional cells are found in other elderly persons, but appear with distinguishing frequency in the brains of those with Alzheimer's. These pathological cells tend to be concentrated in the base of the forebrain as well as throughout the cortical association areas. Cells in this area relay nerve impulses to the cerebral cortex and to the hippocampus which is vital to the formation of memories. The cells affected in these areas rely on the neurotransmitter acetylcholine for communication.

Several hypotheses have been proposed to explain the etiology of Alzheimer's disease, although none are fully supported by available data. One of the most widely accepted is that this disease is caused by viral infection, perhaps by a slow virus, so-called because it takes a very long time following infection for symptoms of disease to develop. Greatest support for this theory comes from the behavioral and pathological resemblance that Alzheimer's disease has to two slow-virus diseases in humans and to one in sheep. Other theories focus on the presence of certain chemicals in the brain. More than 20 years ago, researchers reported elevated levels of aluminum in the brains of Alzheimer's patients but this has been found to be unrelated to factors causing the diseases. Others have suggested that the brains of people with Alzheimer's have lower levels of choline, which is an important building block for both cell membranes and the neurotransmitter acetylcholine, but these results are preliminary. Substantial evidence that Alzheimer's disease may be a genetic disorder has accumulated during the past decade. There is a growing recognition that the disease runs in families and that all patients with Down syndrome, which is caused by a genetic abnormality, develop the brain lesions characteristic of Alzheimer's disease if the patients survive to adulthood. Perhaps information on the extra chromosome 21 as seen most often in Down's syndrome is also responsible for Alzheimer's disease.

Vascular Dementia. A disruption in the blood supply to the brain can cause vascular dementia. This cognitive disorder is caused by a succession of small strokes. Patients with this disorder typically have dozens or hundreds of such strokes over the course of the illness. Many older persons who never receive the diagnosis still experience one or more interruptions of the blood supply to their brain. It is sometimes difficult to distinguish between the dementia associated with Alzheimer's disease and vascular dementia. This differentiation can sometimes be done on the basis of age (since Alzheimer's typically occurs in older persons) and disease course. Alzheimer's generally begins very gradually and its course involves a steady deterioration. The deterioration in intellectual functioning and movement of vascular dementia follows a characteristic pattern of sudden deterioration followed by a period of stability and then another abrupt behavioral deterioration. Partly due to the stepwise character of this disorder, patients in the early stages of vascular dementia are usually well aware of its impact on their ability to work, relate to others, and remain independent. Depression and suicide are understandable accompaniments of this stage of the disease--these patients have been found to be more emotionally impaired than patients with Alzheimer's disease. More than one-third of patients with vascular dementia have more blunted affect, motor retardation, low motivation, unusual thoughts, and somatic concerns.

Treatment and Prevention. Within the last decade, researchers have studied drugs that temporarily reverse the cognitive deficits associated with Alzheimer's disease and vascular dementia. Reports of success using cognitive therapy techniques to remediate memory and cognitive impairments have also appeared in recent years, although these are generally more successful with patients who are younger and have traumatic injuries. Extensive experience has confirmed the importance of social support for persons who are elderly. Even the symptoms of Alzheimer's disease are lessened when patients' needs for care and concern are satisfied.

Other Cognitive Disorders

Substance-Induced Cognitive Disorders. A diagnosis of substance intoxication delirium is made when the cognitive symptoms associated with intoxication (memory impairment, disorientation, or language disturbance) are greater than usual, a disturbance of consciousness that interferes with the clarity of awareness of the environment is observed, and the symptoms of intoxication are severe enough to call for clinical attention. This delirium arises within minutes to hours after ingesting high doses of drugs like cannabis, cocaine, and the hallucinogens. With drugs like alcohol or the barbiturates, several days of intoxication may be required in order for the delirium to develop.

Substance withdrawal delirium develops when tissue and fluid concentrations of the substance in the body decrease suddenly after prolonged, heavy substance ingestion. Depending on the substance involved, substance withdrawal delirium can last for only a few hours or as long as several weeks. Long-term alcohol abusers are at heightened risk for experiencing alcohol withdrawal delirium more familiarly known as delirium tremens which typically begins a week or so after drinking has stopped. This delirium occurs relatively rarely. Symptoms include difficulty attending to environmental stimuli, constant shifts in attention, and disorganized thinking (rambling or irrelevant speech or incoherence). People experiencing delirium tremens can develop vivid visual, auditory, or tactile hallucinations. These individuals may also experience paranoid delusions. Untreated, delirium tremens can be life threatening; these patients can be sedated thereby preventing development of the syndrome.

Substance-induced persisting dementia typically follows a sustained period of heavy substance abuse extending over many years. Its symptoms are those of dementia (impaired ability to learn new information or recall previously learned information, aphasia, apraxia, agnosia, and deficits in planning organizing) and the cognitive deficits must be substantial enough to cause significant impairment in social or occupational functioning and represent a decline from previous levels of functioning. The symptoms persist after substance intoxication or withdrawal has ended. Many people who are homeless have substance-induced persisting dementia.

Substance-induced persisting amnestic disorder is a chronic, profound, irreversible memory disorder cause d by sustained substance abuse. When this serious disorder follows prolonged, heavy alcohol ingestion and the chronic thiamin deficiency that typically accompanies it, it's termed Wernicke-Korsakoff syndrome. Thiamin deficiency happens because alcoholics tend to rely in alcohol which is devoid of vitamins and minerals for most of their calories. Wernicke-Korsakoff syndrome typically begins with an acute, time-limited episode of confusion, balance and coordination problems, eye movement abnormalities, and other signs of neurological disorder. When these symptoms subside, the main feature of the chronic phase remains (profound, irreversible memory impairment). This phase is marked by four principle cognitive deficits: anterograde amnesia, retrograde amnesia, visuoperceptual deficits, and problem-solving deficits.

Treatment and Prevention. Several substances hasten the removal of ethanol from the blood when they're introduced directly into the bloodstream; the most effective is fructose, a naturally occurring fruit sugar. However, none can be taken by mouth because the oral route to the bloodstream causes chemical alteration of the substances as they pass through the gastrointestinal tract. Substance withdrawal delirium can be prevented using a combination of tranquilizing drugs and gradual reduction in the concentration of the abused drug in the blood. If withdrawal cannot be prevented, the agitation, anxiety and hallucinations that accompany it just be treated with substantial doses of tranquilizers and drugs. When left untreated, delirium tremens carries a substantial mortality risk. An innovative program that's designed to teach patients with alcohol-induced persisting amnestic disorder and alcohol-induced persisting dementia how to compensate for their memory impairments has recently been developed. When patients are allowed to practice on a variety of memory tasks; performance was significantly improved.

Cognitive Disorders Due to General Medical Conditions

Infections, tumors, and endocrine, metabolic, and neurological diseases also affect brain function and behavior. Delirium and dementia due to HIV disease are cognitive disorders that can result from infection by the human inmmunodeficiency virus (HIV). Acquired immune deficiency syndrome (AIDS) is a life-threatening physical disease caused by HIV and is sometimes accompanied by cognitive impairment. From 5 to 35% of all persons who become HIV positive ultimately develop dementia due to HIV disease. Common cognitive symptoms at this stage of the dementia include forgetfulness and poor concentration. Later, psychomotor retardation, decreased alertness, apathy, withdrawal, diminished interest in work, and loss of interest in sex may develop. Over the next several months, confusion, disorientation, seizures, mutism, profound dementia,, coma, and death typically ensue. The prevalence of delirium due to :HIV disease is comparable to that of HIV-related dementia and is characterized by feelings of anger, hostility, confusion, denial, hallucinations and delusions, some of which involve paranoia. At present, no effective treatment has been developed to control the effects of HIV on the central nervous system. Drugs are available, however, to ease the agitation, depression, and anxiety associated the this life-threatening disease. The brain disorders that result from HIV infection are preventable by using safe-sex practices and inducing IV drug abuser to stop sharing needles.

The Thinking about Multicultural Issues box on page 538 presents research regarding a series of videotapes aimed at reducing rates of HIV and AIDS among yet another high-risk group: African-American women living in inner-city Chicago.

Dementia due to Huntington's disease is a genetic disorder that is characterized by changes in personality, intellect, memory, interpersonal behavior, and movement, typically culminating in dementia; generally, this disorder begins in mid-life (peak age is 40). This disorder invariably affects those who inherit the gene. It was found that nearly all the people who had this disease in the eastern United States could be traced to about six individuals who had emigrated to this country in 1630 from a tiny village in Suffolk, England. The deteriorating course of the disease ultimately leads to depression, dementia, psychosis, and chorea which is characterized by involuntary, jerky movements of the face, arms, and legs. About 90% of Huntington's patients ultimately develop dementia during the course of their illness; about 40% become clinically depressed. Suicide is common among two groups those who have the potential to develop the disorder and those who have acquired it. At present, Huntington's disease in incurable. Treatment is largely supportive; it consists of drugs to control chorea and combat depression. No effective treatment exists for Huntington-induced dementia. Prevention begins with genetic counseling of persons with family histories of the disorder.

Dementia due to Parkinson's disease. Parkinson's disease is caused by the destruction of brain cells that produce the neurotransmitter dopamine. The resulting dopamine deficiency results in a degenerative process that involves tremor, muscular rigidity, bradykinesia (exaggeratedly slow movement because of muscle rigidity), stooped posture, and a shuffling gait. The age of onset is between 40 and 60 and, although the etiology is often unknown, the disorder can be caused by encephalitis, carbon monoxide poisoning, or head injury. Parkinson's-like symptoms can also be caused by the long-term use of major tranquilizing drugs, such as those used to treat schizophrenia. Depression and dementia are quite common in Parkinson's disease. Depression affects 50 to 90% of these patients, and dementia affect 25 to 50%. Some evidence suggests that dementia is more common among individuals who develop Parkinson's disease late in life. The drug L-dopa (a precursor of dopamine) is given to Parkinson's patients to increase the level of dopamine in the brain. However, L-dopa has significant mental side effects, including confusion and agitation.

Epilepsy is a chronic neurological syndrome characterized by repeated and recurrent seizures. A seizure is a pathophysiological brain disturbance caused by the spontaneous, excessive discharge of neurons in the cortex. A seizure may involve abnormal movement or cessation of movement; an unusual smell, taste, or sight; a behavioral disturbance; or a change in state of consciousness. Almost any disturbance to the brain can cause epilepsy, hence the name syndrome rather than disorder. Epileptic seizures can occur at any time and are clearly provoked by stress in certain individuals. Some people with seizure disorders experience several seizures a day, whereas others may have one every few months or less. Grand mal epilepsy is one of the most common seizure disorders and involves loss of consciousness and a generalized convulsion of the entire body. Petit mal epilepsy involves a brief disruption in consciousness, generally lasting form 2 to 10 seconds, which may be overlooked by observers. The patient may stare vacantly, with the mouth open and the eyes blinking or turning up. Jacksonian seizures are signaled by a variety of partial motor symptoms. Initially, these symptoms involve the involuntary movement of a finger or a toe; ultimately, they lead to a period of involuntary jerking of a part of one entire side of the body. Jacksonian seizures typically last from 20 to 30 seconds. Temporal lobe epilepsy may lead the individual to perform unusual behavior and may involve episodic violence during the period of attack.

Personality disturbances are the most common psychiatric complication of epilepsy. Symptoms are varied, including changes in sexual behavior, and increased preoccupation with religion, heightened experience of emotions, and changes in conversation. Psychosis has also been reported in temporal lobe epileptics between seizures. The advent of antiepileptic drugs in recent decades have resulted in helping 75% of individuals with epilepsy experience either complete or substantial remission of seizures. Surgical removal of the diseased portion of the brain responsible for the seizure disorder is another treatment option. However, use of antiepileptic drugs is the treatment of choice.

KEY IDEAS AND OBJECTIVES FOR STUDENTS

After reading the chapter, you should be able to answer each of the following questions:

1. How have changes in life expectancy affected interest in and study of the elderly? Are supposedly inevitable features of aging preventable?

2. Which cognitive disorders are acute and reversible? Which cognitive disorders are chronic and irreversible? Which cognitive disorders involve persisting amnesia that is characterized by a profound, irreversible disturbance in memory?

3. What are the symptoms and characteristics of Alzheimer's disease?

4. What are the characteristics of vascular dementia? Are effective treatments available?

5. What are the substance-induced conditions?

6. What are the characteristics of cognitive disorders due to general medical conditions? Which diseases are included in this category? How effective is treatment?

Cognitive Disorders in the Movies

1. On Golden Pond (1981, Family Home Entertainment, 109 min). Henry Fonda and Katherine Hepburn star in this film about an elderly couple trying to enjoy what may be their last summer together. The plot focuses on family conflicts particularly between the father (Henry Fonda) and daughter (Jane Fonda).

Questions after watching the movie.

1. How are this elderly couple similar (or different) from other elderly adults that you know?

2. Does the film's portrayal of aging match what you learned from the text? How could the film have better dealt with the aging issues?

Using Case Studies in Abnormal Behavior by Meyer and Osborne:
Organic Mental Disorders

General Summary

Chapter 15 focuses primarily on Cognitive Disorders. Case material is presented for three individuals: (a) a child who had a large portion of his brain removed, (b) an individual with a mood disorder due to brain trauma, and (c) an individual with Alzheimer's disease.

Case Comparisons

Recovery of function: The Case of Harry. This example is not a clear diagnostic problem. Rather the case shows the ability of the brain to recover from an injury. Harry had a large portion of his brain removed when he was 5 years old. At 15 and 21 years after surgery he was performing in the high average range of intelligence with a verbal IQ score in the superior range.

Affective Syndrome Resulting from Brain Trauma: The Case of Bjorn. This case illustrates the extent with which organic factors can results in changes in mood. The case material presented does not allow for a diagnosis of Mood Disorder due to a General Medical Condition, however, clearly Bjorn has many of the symptoms of depression that appear to be the result of his injury. After reading the case, you should be able to discuss the similarities and differences between this type of mood disorder and other mood disorders discussed in Chapter 7. What treatment options were considered for this case? Which was used?

Alzheimer's Disease: The Case of Al. The diagnostic criteria for dementia of the Alzheimer's type are presented on pages 524-526 of the text. Provide a summary of the specific characteristics of Al that support the diagnosis. Are any of the criteria questionable? What factors may have led to the development of this problem for Al? What treatment options were considered? Which were used?

<u>Integrating Perspectives</u>
A Biopsychosocial Model

The Case of Bjorn

<u>Biological Factors</u>

•Bjorn had clear brain trauma. His skull was fractured and there were sever contusions to the underlying brain tissue. He has seizures during recovery.

<u>Psychological Factors</u>

•Clear psychological changes were noted, but it is appears that these changes were the result, not the cause of the problem.

•Bjorn's premorbid adjustment (he was highly sociable and quite active in campus activities) helped identify the existence of a problem.

•He used memorization strategies that he had learned and practiced early in college to counter some of the deficits that the injury caused.

<u>Social Factors</u>

•The strength of his family and friendships helped identify the existence of the problem, but also served to reinforce his passivity and unresponsiveness.

Sample Multiple-Choice Questions

1. Which is NOT a reason for why the U.S. population is aging so rapidly?
   a. people are having fewer children
   b. the increase of affordable health care for the elderly
   c. society's growing concern for better nutrition and exercise
   d. medicine advances

2. Ms. Powell is a 69-year-old college professor who wants to know if her increased forgetting is normal. ____________ is the term for the normal impact of the aging process on thinking, problem-solving, and remembering.
   a. Senility
   b. Dementia
   c. Alzheimer's disease
   d. Normal cognitive aging

3. Barry is a 33-year-old man diagnosed with the AIDS virus. Because of his illness, he has experienced a number of high fevers and brain damage. Soon after his 33rd birthday, Barry experienced a loss in memory and global deterioration in his intellectual, emotional, and cognitive abilities. He has great difficulty performing tasks that requires him to remember, learn, or use facts. Occasionally, he has bouts of depression and paranoid thinking. Barry has ____________.
   a. delirium
   b. dementia
   c. Alzheimer's disease
   d. amnestic disorder

4. Amy is a 6-year-old with influenza. She has had a high fever for over three days. On the days she had the fever, she experienced some disorientation, and had difficulty paying attention. These symptoms disappeared when her temperature returned to normal. Amy experienced a(n) ______________.
   a. chronic cognitive disorder
   b. episode of dementia
   c. acute cognitive disorder
   d. episode of amnesia

5. The prevalence of Alzheimer's disease in the U.S. among persons over 65 years of age is approximately _______ percent.
   a. 10
   b. 25
   c. 45
   d. 75

6. Martha has memory problems associated with her Alzheimer's disease. She has decreased retention time and forgets important information. She also tends to distort the recall of events in the form of confabulations. Her memory problems tend to be accompanied by disorientation to place, time, and person. She has __________ forgetfulness.
   a. malignant
   b. demented
   c. senile
   d. benign

7. Which of the following is TRUE about drugs that reduce the effects of dementia?
   a. No such drugs exist.
   b. Drugs exist which can permanently reverse the effects of dementia.
   c. The best drugs available for reducing the effects of dementia are antidepressants.
   d. Drugs that are cable of restoring the damaged regions of the brain are being developed, but it will be a long and arduous process.

8. Janet is a long-term alcohol abuser. She is particularly high at risk for experiencing alcohol withdrawal delirium, or ___________.
   a. substance intoxication delirium
   b. delirium tremens
   c. substance induced dementia
   d. substance induced amnesia

9. Approximately __________ percent of persons who are HIV positive develop dementia due to HIV disease.
   a. 1-5
   b. 5-10
   c. 5-35
   d. 35-50

10. Lorenzo has been diagnosed with Parkinson's disease. His doctor will most likely prescribe ___________ in order to help alleviate the movement disorders associated with this disease.
   a. anticonvulsants
   b. antidepressants
   c. antiepileptics
   d. L-Dopa

Answer Key

1. b
2. d
3. b
4. c
5. a
6. a
7. d
8. b
9. c
10. d

Chapter 17 VIOLENCE

Description

Abuse can take many forms (physical, emotional, or sexual). Physical abuse toward a partner or child refers to acts of physical aggression by one individual against the other (e.g., slapping, hitting, kicking, biting, and beating). With adult partners, repeated acts of physical aggression and/or physical aggression against another adult leading to fear of the partner is abuse. Physical abuse of children refers to physical aggression that has injurious effects on a child. Definitions of rape vary somewhat across states, but rape generally refers to unwanted or non-consensual sexual activity that is forced or coerced against another. DSM-IV includes a new category, "Problems Related to Abuse or Neglect," which includes physical abuse of a child, sexual abuse of a child, physical abuse of an adult, and sexual abuse of an adult.

Partner Abuse

According to DSM-IV, partner abuse refers to acts of physical aggression such as slapping, pushing, shoving, and kicking that occur more than once per year. It also refers to acts of physical aggression that result in physical injury requiring medical attention and can include physically aggressive acts involving threats and intimidation. About one third of all married women will be victims of some form of physical aggression during their lifetime, and 10% will be victims of severe and repeated violence. Every year, approximately 12% of married women are victims of some act of physical aggression; about 4% are victims of violence that takes the form of beating, threatening with or using a knife or gun. About 2,000 women are killed in the U.S. each year.

Although rates of physical aggression by men and women are roughly equal, women clearly experience more injuries than men. In couples in which women are severely abused and often injured, physical aggression by men is usually much more common than physical aggression by women, and when women engage in physical aggression it is generally in self-defense. It appears that rates of physical aggression within marriage differ according to age, education, race, and social class. Physical aggression decreases with age, with men and women in their twenties most likely to be in physically abusive relationships. In addition, African American men are more likely to engage in physical aggression than White men. However, higher rates of physical aggression in Blacks were found only among lower-income respondents. The Thinking About Multicultural Issues box on page 546 addresses racial and SES differences in rates of abuse in more detail. While higher rates of physical aggression are reported among those with less education and less income, child abuse, partner abuse, and elder abuse occur in all socioeconomic classes. Risk of all three forms of abuse is higher among those who are poor and who hold low prestige jobs.

Rape

Definitions of rape vary somewhat across states, but rape generally refers to unwanted or non-consensual sexual activity that is forced or coerced against another individual. Most rape victims are young. In fact, a national survey revealed that 29% of rape victims were under

11 years old, 32% were between ages 11 and 17, and another 22% between ages 18 and 24. In close to 80% of cases, the woman knows the rapist. The most likely known person to rape is an acquaintance (29%) followed next by a relative (16%). Approximately 9% of women reported being raped by former or current husbands. A national survey of rape and sexual aggression showed the extent of sexual aggression on college campuses: 28% of college women reported experiencing rape or attempted rape since age 14 and 54% reported some form of sexual victimization. Men are also victims of rape; it is estimated that 1%-3% of inmates are sexually assaulted. Marital rape has only recently been legally recognized; approximately 3-14% of married women report being raped by their husbands.

Acquaintance Rape. Date rape is the most common form of acquaintance rape and involves unwanted or nonconsensual sexual activity that is forced or coerced against a person by her dating partner. Defining consent to sexual activity is controversial, and males and females differ in their perceptions of situations which constitute rape (see Table 17.1 on page 550).

The Impact of Rape. Whether they resist or not, women who are raped are frequently beaten. Women who have been raped report more medical problems than those who have not been raped. Posttraumatic stress disorder frequently develops: 94% meet criteria one week after the rape; 47% meet criteria after 3 months.

Child Abuse

While physical and sexual abuse are the most commonly discussed forms of child abuse, the most prevalent form of abuse is neglect, or inadequate supervision and lack of attention to the physical and emotional needs of the child. Another infrequently discussed form of abuse is emotional abuse which generally refers to being harsh, critical, and overly demanding of the child. About half of all child abuse is neglect; approximately 25% is physical abuse, roughly 15% involve sexual abuse, and about 10% involve emotional abuse. There are no specific behaviors that define child abuse or neglect. However, physical abuse refers to non-accidental injuries as a result of acts of commission or omission by caretakers. Neglect refers to the failure of a parent to provide minimal standards of care and support for children. About 10% of parents display violent behavior toward their children (based on a national sample), and 1,100 children died in 1992 from abuse or neglect. When all types of abuse are considered, the natural parents are the most likely individuals to be charged with child maltreatment. However, other caregivers (step-parents, foster parents, relatives) are more likely to sexually abuse children than parents. Women are reported for child abuse more than men, but risk of injury is much higher when the abuser is male.

The Impact of Child Abuse. Being the victim of physical abuse as a child increases the likelihood that the child will later engage in violent and/or abusive behaviors. The probability of intergenerational transmission of violence increases as the exposure to different types of violence increases. However, it is important to note that most abused children do not grow up to abuse their own children. In addition to the transmission of abuse which may occur across generations, there are often immediate and deleterious consequences to the child who has been victimized. Victims of child physical and sexual abuse have higher rates of attempted and completed suicides than others; risk of suicide increases with repeated abuse. Consequences of severe physical or sexual abuse in childhood include: three times the risk of drug and alcohol abuse as the general population; anxiety symptoms in the form of posttraumatic stress disorder; and more academic problems than nonabused children.

Causes

Partner Abuse

There are three perspectives on the causes of partner abuse: feminist, psychological and biological.

Feminist Accounts. The major tenet of the feminist accounts of physical abuse is that men use their power to gain control over women, which is condoned both implicitly and explicitly, by society.

Psychological Explanations. Two psychological explanations of partner abuse predominate: 1) individual psychopathology of those involved in the physically abusive relationship; and 2) the dyadic interactions between the husband and wife that lead to a physically abusive act. These two perspectives are not mutually exclusive. Individual explanations of women's behavior initially focused on the women's self-destructive, masochistic behavior (1970s). Blaming the woman for the abuse she suffered is no longer accepted. Today, the focus has shifted to the effects the woman may have suffered as a result of the abuse. About 35-45% of physically abused women receive a PTSD diagnosis, with higher rates among women who seek refuge in a shelter. Major depression and drug or alcohol abuse may also result. Individual explanations of men's behavior have focused on the fact that physically abusive men tend to score in the pathological range on scales relating to aggressiveness and having a negativistic style of interacting. Further, there is increasing agreement that individuals who engage in minor and isolated acts of physical aggression are quite different from those who engage in repeated and severe acts of aggression against their partners. Alcohol use is associated with husband to wife aggression. However, alcohol is used at the time of a physically aggressive incident in only 24% of the cases. Alcohol alone is not a necessary or sufficient condition for the expression of physical aggression against a partner. Relationship explanations have concluded that the interactions between the husband and wife are central in the escalation pattern of which physical aggression is the final result. Communication patterns of men and women in physically abusive relationships are different from those in non-abusive relationships.

Biological Explanations. There is accumulating evidence that biological factors may contribute to physical aggression against a spouse. Five biological variables often implicated in the development of partner abuse are brain injury, testosterone, physiological reactivity, evolutionary analyses, and genetic factors. Brain injury in men has been associated with reports of outbursts of rage, irritability, and reduced impulse control; 61% of men attending court ordered treatment to decrease battering of their partners had experienced significant head injury. Testosterone levels are 10 times higher in males than in females. Castration reduces aggression in a variety of male animals, and testosterone injections reinstate the aggression. However, research indicates that the relationship between testosterone and aggression is weak and only suggests a relationship. Physiological reactivity of physically abusive men has been examined, but physically abusive men do not appear to differ from maritally discordant non-abusive men. However, about 20% of physically abusive men had heart rates which declined while in a heated discussion with their partner about a marital problem. These men were also seen as probably unamenable to treatment and similar to psychopaths in their physiological responding.

Evolutionary factors have been examined to account for aggressive behavior. Daly and Wilson (1988) hypothesized that men and women attempt to maximize their gene potential; this is consistent with the fact that men and women kill their step children more frequently than they kill their own children. Also, since jealousy is the leading motive in spousal homicide, males may be acting to protect their own gene pool from being "mixed" with others. While these are consistent with an evolutionary view, there are other possible interpretations of these data. Genetic factors have been examined for several decades. According to animal behaviorists, some differences in aggressive behavior can be ascribed to genetic differences; however, the role of genes in the aggressive behavior of humans is small compared to that of environment.

Rape

Feminist Accounts. Susan Brownmiller (1975) proposed an influential feminist view of rape that focuses on rape as a weapon to generate fear and intimidation to control women. This view of rape as violent behavior is consistent with the fact that rapists are much more likely to have a history of nonsexual criminal and aggressive activity than non-rapists. A large proportion of adolescent sex offenders, particularly rapists, also have a history of conduct disorder.

Rape as Deviant Sexual Arousal? This perspective views rape as a paraphilia or arousal to deviant acts (use of force or humiliation). A number of studies that have shown that rapists' sexual arousal patterns differ from those of non-rapists. Rapists demonstrate more sexual arousal to rape stories than nonrapists. Attempts to replicate these findings, however, have often failed. Other evidence supports the view that rape is motivated by normal sexual urges.

Portrayals of Violent Pornography. Teenagers commit a disproportionately large number of rapes and other forms of sexual violence. Antipornography groups claim one factor contributing to rape is the explicit association between sex and violence in movies, rock videos, and music lyrics. Research suggest that repeated exposure to violent pornography might reduce the likelihood of a man responding appropriately when the woman indicates that she does not consent to sex.

Miscommunication or Provocation? Sexual scripts in which men are expected to pursue sex, women are expected to resist men overcome the women's resistance are common. This has led some to conceptualize date rape a form of miscommunication rather than sexual violence.

Child Abuse

The factors that lead to partner/wife abuse and the factors that lead to child abuse have clear similarities. Men who abuse their children are more likely to abuse their wives than are men who do not abuse their children. On the other hand, many adults engage in abusive behavior toward their children but do not engage in abusive behavior toward their partners.

Poverty. Child abuse occurs in all socioeconomic levels but is most common among individuals who are poor. Wolfe found that 48% of parents charged with neglect were receiving public assistance, and 34% of parents charged with physical abuse were receiving public assistance. Poverty is disproportionately represented across racial groups in the United States. Approximately 39% of Hispanic children, 45% of African American children, and 15% of white children live in poverty. Children in families maintained by a woman with no husband present are most likely to be living in poverty. This also varies by race/ethnicity: 54% of African-American children live with a single parent compared to 30% for Hispanic children and 19% for White children.

Age of Caregiver. Young mothers are at greatest risk for abusing their children. Young, single mothers lacking in family and social support are at greatest risk.

Caregiver Psychopathology. Abusive individuals are impulsive, have trouble with anger control, and mothers at risk for severely injuring their children are very dissatisfied with their marriages or cohabiting relationships and are depressed. Parents who abuse alcohol and drugs are more likely to abuse their children than parents who do not abuse these substances.

Caregiver History of Being Abused As a Child. Parents who abuse their children are more likely to have been abused themselves than parents who do not abuse their children. However, most abused children do not grow up to be abusers.

Unrealistic Expectations of Children. Abusive parents overestimate their children's abilities to take care of themselves, to wait patiently, and to behave properly. This may lead parents to get angry at their children and become physically abusive when expectations are not met.

Child Factors. Parents are most likely to abuse children who are less than four years old. Teenagers are the next most likely age group to be abused and neglected. Children with irregular sleeping patterns, poor eating habits, and/or oppositional, hyperactive or conduct disordered behavior are at greater risk for abuse.

Treatment

Partner Abuse

Treatment for problems of partner abuse can involve the wife, the husband, or both. Usually women receive shelter and counseling aimed at decreasing self-blame for the physical abuse, at evaluating the marriage as it is, and providing alternatives to the marriage.

Treatment for abusive husbands is usually a group format with the goals of reducing both the physical and psychological aggression in the marriage. Taking full responsibility for the physical aggression against the wife -no matter what the provocation by the wife is reported to be-is a key first goal of intervention. Couples treatment is relatively new, and may focus on anger control techniques. The format is designed for couples who want to stay together, for couples in which the wife is not fearful of her husband and the level of aggression has not merited attention. It is geared towards the very large number of couples who engage in lower levels of physical aggression and who attend clinics throughout the country. Emphasis is placed on how each partner contributes to the escalation of the physical aggression, on each partner's responsibility for his/her physical aggression, on increasing communication and enabling each partner to better express his/her feelings without name-calling, cataloging past wrongs, and labeling of the partner (you are crazy, lazy or an evil person). It is also accomplished by encouraging both the husband and wife to help understand what the "real" problems are that contribute to the conflict escalation resulting sometimes in partner violence. Both individual treatment programs for men and women and couples treatment have been effective.

Rape

It has been estimated that between 50 and 75% of all jailed sex offenders get no treatment at all. One third of all inmates offered treatment refuse it. Even when the most effective treatment techniques are implemented, long-term results are unclear or significant but small. Relapse rates vary from 3-31%, depending on length of follow-up, and rapists relapse more often than other paraphiliacs. The most violent and dangerous individuals are the least likely to benefit from treatment. Violent rapists are very likely to repeat their crimes when released from prison. The lack of effective treatments is related to the movement to keep the public informed of identified sex offenders (see page 556) and the Sexually Violent Predators Law in the state of Washington which allows involuntary civil confinement of dangerous sex offenders after completion of prison sentences.

Treatment for rape victims includes group and support therapy, exposure and anxiety management approaches, which may change or restructure beliefs that are detrimental to the woman's functioning.

Child Abuse

Parents Anonymous (PA). This is a volunteer program modeled after Alcoholics Anonymous. Parent training for parents with problems in parenting but who have not actually become physically abusive can result in decreased use of punishment, increased use of positive reinforcement and constructive parenting styles. However, such changes are often not maintained across time. Low income was found to be the biggest predictor of poor response to treatment for parenting problems. Discord between partners and depression are also associated with parenting problems. Effective treatment must consider parents in their total environment and the stresses they cope with.

Since physically abused children are at risk for having social skills deficits and problems with anxiety, anger and aggression, treatment of the child is often warranted. Unfortunately, there is very little systematic research regarding the effectiveness of such treatment programs.

KEY IDEAS AND OBJECTIVES FOR STUDENTS

After reading the chapter, you should be able to answer each of the following questions:

1. What is the prevalence of physical aggression in relationships, including abuse and severe battering? Are men or women more likely to be injured in aggressive relationships?

2. What is the prevalence of rape? How does this vary by age and by knowledge of the attacker?

3. Who is more likely to physically abuse their children, mothers or fathers? Who is more likely to cause injury?

4. What are the potential causes of violence towards women? What factors are associated with being physically violent towards one's partner as an adult?

5. What factors are associated with the cause of rape?

6. What are the risk factors for child abuse?

7. What ages of children are most likely to be physically abused by their parents?

8. What is the first priority for women who have been battered ?

9. What treatments are available for women and their partners who have been abusive? For whom are these treatments effective?

10. What treatment is typically received by convicted rapists and other sexual offenders? Is treatment effective?

11. What type of treatment is used with rape victims?

12. What treatments are provided for abusive parents? Are they effective?

Violence in the Movies

1. Sleeping With the Enemy (1991, Fox Video, 99 min). This movie illustrates repetitive and severe domestic violence, including emotional, physical and sexual abuse. Since the couple portrayed in the film is of high SES, it demonstrates the fact that domestic violence occurs at all SES levels. The character played by Julia Roberts is subject to efforts at extreme control by her husband, who demands perfection (e.g., cans on the shelves lined up properly, towels hanging in a straight line on the towel rack) and limited contact with other people. After faking her own death to escape her husband and establishing a new life in another location, Julia Roberts is able to return to some semblance of normal living. The film ends with a confrontation with her husband when he discovers her whereabouts. Although the film is fairly dramatic, it does convey the severity of abuse many women experience.

Questions watching the movie:

1. Given the text's description of the characteristics of men who abuse their partners, how well did the movie do in presenting an accurate portrayal of an abusive husband? What "errors" (including errors of omission and commission) were made?

2. How well did the movie do in presenting the effects of the abuse on the abused wife? What "errors" (including errors of omission and commission) were made?

3. How did the film deal with the etiology of this abusive relationship? What were the major consistencies (or inconsistencies) with contemporary theories?

4. Although this film ended with the death of the abusive husband, what treatments would you recommend for this character?

5. If you were to be a consultant on a "remake" of this film, what advice would you give the director to help make the symptoms, etiology, and treatment more contemporary?

2. The Accused (1988, Paramount Home Video, 110 min) This film deals with the brutal rape of a young woman by multiple men at a bar. The film demonstrates the way in which rape victims are often blamed for their victimization, and are evaluated on the basis of their dress, behavior, use of alcohol, and previous history. The perspectives of the victim, played by Jodie Foster, a female assistant district attorney who prosecutes her case (played by Kelly McGillis), the perpetrators, other male lawyers, and the male-dominated legal system are explored. Students could focus on issues of consent and gender differences after watching this movie.

Questions after watching the movie:

1. Given the text's description of the characteristics of rapists, how well did the perpetrators in this film match these characteristics? What were the differences between the characters in the movie and the description in the text?

2. How did the film address the reasons for the rape? Which theories fit best with the film? Which theories are inconsistent?

3. Using Table 17.1 on page 550 of the text as a model, was this rape the result (or partly the result) of miscommunication and differences between men's and women's perceptions of consent?

4. Which theory or theories can explain the behavior of the men who did not have forced sexual intercourse with the character portrayed by Jodie Foster, but who cheered on those men who did?

5. What recommendations would you make to change societal attitudes about rape?

6. If you were to be a consultant for a "remake" of this film, what advice would you give the director to help make the symptoms, etiology, and treatment more contemporary?

Using Case Studies in Abnormal Psychology by Meyer & Osborne:
Disorders with Violence

Chapter 13, Disorders with Violence, of the casebook focuses on multiple types of violence. The chapter opens with the case of Jack Ruby, who killed Lee Harvey Oswald (who assassinated President John F. Kennedy). His life is explored in the context of several causal models, including social psychology theories, organic/biological/genetic theories, affective disorder theory, and psychopathy-antisocial personality disorder theory. Different treatments are briefly reviewed from the perspective of causal models. The difficulty in accurately predicting violence is also discussed. Family violence is illustrated through two cases, one involving physical abuse and one involving sexual abuse of a child. Risk factors for family violence and treatment options are covered at the close of the chapter. Note: Other cases from this book which involve violence can be found in the following: Chapter 1 - O. J. Simpson (chapter 1 of the IRM); Chapter 7 - Joseph Westbecker (chapter 7 of the IRM); Chapter 8 - Jeffrey Dahmer (chapter 8 of the IRM); Chapter 11 - Ted Bundy (chapter 12 of the IRM); and Chapter 16 - John Hinckley (chapter 21 of the IRM).

Case Comparisons

Causes of Violence: The Case of Jack Ruby. Jack Ruby, who died in prison after killing Lee Harvey Oswald, was exposed to many factors which have been linked to aggressive and violent behavior. These factors include: family history of significant pathology, childhood conduct disordered behavior and criminal activity, physical abuse suffered as a child, and adult antisocial behavior. Given what you know about specific diagnoses and personality disorders, what evidence is there to suggest that Jack Ruby suffered from an Axis I disorder? Be sure to identify the specific disorders which should be considered and specific examples of behavior which support a diagnosis. What evidence suggests an Axis II disorder? Be sure to identify the specific personality disorder(s) to be considered and examples which support your conclusion. If Jack Ruby had sought treatment as an adult, what treatments would have been appropriate?

Child Sexual Abuse: The Case of Charles. Charles sexually abused his 8-year-old daughter, Vicki over a six-month period. The case describes a marriage that gradually deteriorated, the development of alcoholism in Charles' wife, and the discovery by a neighbor of the sexual abuse. Based on the description, do you think that Charles exhibited any specific DSM-IV diagnosis? Which one(s)? Support your answer with specific examples. Which theoretical models presented in the text would best explain the cause of the abuse? Although the casebook does not describe the treatment Charles received, what characteristics would likely be included in successful treatment? What do you think were the effects on Vicki of having been abused?

Child Physical Abuse: The Case of Abby. Abby displayed several characteristics described in the text that have been identified as risk factors for becoming an abusive parent. Provide a summary of the risk factors, giving specific examples. What risk factors were not displayed by Abby? What factors led to the greater likelihood of abusing her son, rather than her daughter? Did Abby exhibit any characteristics of a DSM-IV Axis I or Axis II disorder?

Which one(s)? Support your answer with specific answers. Although Abby made some gains in treatment, she terminated prematurely. What suggestions do you have for making treatment more successful for parents like Abby? What do you think the effects of being abused will be for her son?

Integrating Perspectives
A Biopsychosocial Model

The Case of Charles

Biological Factors

- Biological factors seemed to not play a major role. Charles acted on natural sexual urges with an inappropriate partner, his daughter.

Psychological Factors

- Charles had a poor relationship with his wife. They rarely had sexual or emotional encounters.
- Charles had always been close to his daughter. They frequently spent time together before she went to bed.
- His first sexual act with his daughter seemed to break down any inhibitions and he quickly progressed from being aroused near her to oral and attempts at vaginal intercourse.

Social Factors

- Child abuse is unacceptable by our society. Even more, incest. This behavior is likely to have lasting effects on both the father and daughter. It resulted in divorce and will likely have profound effects on this child.

Sample Multiple-Choice Questions

1. In a national survey of women, what percentage of married or cohabiting women experience some act of physical aggression against them every year?
   a. 12 percent
   b. 50 percent
   c. 67 percent
   d. 94 percent

2. What percentage of women knew the person who raped them?
   a. 10 percent
   b. 25 percent
   c. 50 percent
   d. 80 percent

3. Mary is a young mother who reports that she often looses her temper. She does not know how to make her 2 year old daughter stop crying, so spanks her child so much that the child cowers in the corner of the room. Her daughter was recently taken to the emergency room where it was learned that she had a dislocated jaw. This behavior can be labeled as
   a. Child Sexual Abuse.
   b. Child Physical Abuse.
   c. Child Neglect.
   d. Child Mistreatment.

4. Nancy was severely abused by her husband for 15 years. She finally ran away and went to a shelter for battered women. During the initial interview, a psychologist noted that she appeared to have symptoms of a psychiatric condition. Which of the following disorders is most likely to have matched her symptoms?
   a. Posttraumatic Stress Disorder.
   b. Borderline Personality Disorder.
   c. Dissociative Identity Disorder.
   d. Antisocial Personality Disorder.

5. Jerry is a 26 year old man who was convicted to raping 13 women over a 4 year period. Jerry describes the events as tremendously more sexually exciting than having sex with a consenting woman. Jerry illustrates which explanation of why men rape?
   a. Rapists need to feel superior to women.
   b. Rape is really a paraphilia.
   c. Rape is the result of men watching pornography.
   d. Rapist feel inferior to women and do not get with traditional sexual interactions.

6. A large percentage of families where the parent is charged with neglect are
   a. upper class, wealthy families.
   b. blue color families.
   c. families were the parent receives public aid.
   d. families with conservative religious beliefs.

7 Parents are most likely to abuse
   a. children under 4 years of age.
   b. teenagers.
   c. young adults over 18 years of age.
   d. older children who act immature.

8. What is the primary issue that the therapist must address in the treatment of abusive couples?
   a. Which spouse is responsible for payment of services.
   b. Which spouse is the cause of the problem.
   c. The safety of the woman.
   d. The health of the woman.

9. Which of the following are the most common treatment approaches for couples involved in partner abuser?
   a. Group treatment for women, no treatment for men.
   b. Group treatment for men, no treatment for women.
   c. Group treatment with separate groups for the women and men.
   d. Group treatment with both men and women present.

10. When are most rapist are most likely to receive treatment?
   a. as an outpatient.
   b. while in prison.
   c. after being released from prison.
   d. most rapist do not receive treatment.

Answer Key

1. a
2. d
3. b
4. a
5. b
6. c
7. a
8. c
9. c
10. d

CHAPTER 18 INDIVIDUAL PSYCHOLOGICAL THERAPIES

Psychoanalysis and Psychodynamic Therapies

Psychoanalysis originated with Freud's work and was the predominant approach in U.S. psychiatry from the mid-1930s until the 1970s. Classic psychoanalysis is intensive treatment (4+ sessions/week) that lasts several years; its lengthy nature and high cost make it an infrequent choice today for most people. Psychotherapies based on psychoanalytic principles vary in content and structure, but share the following concepts: 1) all are concerned with explaining motives behind people's thoughts, feelings, and behaviors; 2) all assume that early childhood experiences determine personality development and subsequent clinical disorders result from early parent-child interactions; 3) all recognize the conflict between opposing psychological forces as an inevitable part of human development, including one's identity as a biological/instinctual animal versus a social being, and those between one's conscious and unconscious motives; 4) all suggest that motives behind behavior are mainly unconscious, which remain hidden via defense mechanisms because they are too threatening or unacceptable; and 5) all suggest that a critical feature is the establishment and development of a special relationship between the patient and therapist.

Psychoanalytic Concepts and Techniques. Free association involves encouraging patients to talk about whatever thoughts or feelings they are experiencing without any effort to censor; this allows for the exploration of a patient's unconscious motives. Resistance is an unwillingness on the part of the patient to cooperate fully in therapy resulting from an unconscious wish to resist personal change. Avoidance of certain topics, disagreeing with the therapist, and arriving late for or missing appointments may occur despite patient's conscious desire to cooperate with treatment. Noting characteristic defenses in response to threatening topics can point to unconscious conflicts experienced by the patient. Transference describes the relationship that develops between the patient and therapist in which the patient responds to the patient in a similar to the way in which he/she responded to significant people in his/her childhood. This leads to unconscious reexperiencing of repressed childhood conflicts. Transference is facilitated by the therapist remaining neutral and nonjudgmental towards patients. Interpretation and denial follow from the development of transference. The therapist shifts from a passive role to a more confrontive one in which interpretations are presented to the patient. Dream interpretation involves exploring the unconscious significance of the patient's dreams and its relationship to current problems. The manifest content refers to what is consciously remembered by the patient and the latent content is the hidden expression of unconscious processes found in dreams. Insight is the goal of all psychoanalytic therapies; this refers to the patient's awareness of unconscious conflicts and psychological defenses, which should lead to more adaptive behaviors.

Neo-Freudian Therapies. Carl Jung broke ranks with Freud and developed analytic psychology. This approach rejects Freud's view that sexuality is the fundamental source of human motivation. Jung believed that sexuality was merely one form of general psychic energy, and he focused on normal and abnormal adult development. He has been considered as a forerunner of humanistic psychology. Alfred Adler also rejected Freud's emphasis on sexuality and had a more optimistic view of human development than Freud. He emphasized the self, a subjective sense of personal worth or adequacy, and the social context of behavior. Basic mistakes referred to Adler's view that maladaptive personal beliefs could lead to psychological problems (e.g., overgeneralizations, impossible goals, etc.). Harry Stack Sullivan emphasized the interpersonal nature of psychological disorders. Parataxic distortions are the effects that problematic interpersonal relationships in childhood have on the adult's misperceptions of reality. He also introduced the concept of the participant observer; he believed that the patient's behavior during therapy sessions was the result of past experience and personality, and of the therapist's subtle influence as a participant in therapy. Sullivan thought that the therapist should be more directive and focused on events in the here and now.

The ego-analytic therapies extended the neo-Freudians' emphasis on the individual's interactions with his/her environment. Greater value was placed on current life circumstances and people's ability to adapt to and control their environments, which are ego functions. Erik Erikson proposed a series of eight psychosocial stages across the lifespan, in which sociocultural reality challenges the person. Heinz Kohut developed self-psychology, in which problems early in life between the mother and child lead to low self-esteem, which causes the child to grow up trying to compensate for feelings of vulnerability through unrealistic and narcissistic striving for love and approval from others. Therapy restores the sense of self through providing acceptance of the patient.

Brief Psychodynamic Therapies. These therapies involve up to 50 hours of treatment, which is considerably shorter than traditional psychodynamic therapy. This approach is appropriate for those patients with strong ego resources, whose problems had acute onset with previous high functioning and adjustment. Treatment goals involve resolving the core conflict (not necessarily changing the personality) through an active and directive therapist. A therapeutic alliance is used to foster the patient's involvement and collaboration in treatment.

An Evaluation of Psychoanalytic Therapies. The popularity of psychoanalytic theory can be linked to: the breadth of the theory, which spans the full range of normal and abnormal behavior; and the extensive explanation of motives behind behavior. Criticisms of the theory include the skepticism with which some of the concepts are viewed (e.g., agoraphobic anxiety about leaving home being related to unconscious to become a prostitute). Another criticism involves the lack of scientific validity and the reliance on the individual patient's success to prove the theory and its value. Two types of research are currently conducted with this theory. Process research is designed to uncover why a particular treatment method has certain effects; it does this by studying the therapist and patient interactions. Outcome research evaluates the effectiveness of treatment. Little outcome research has been conducted with psychoanalytic treatment, with the exception of brief psychodynamic therapy (which has shown promise).

Interpersonal Psychotherapy (IPT)

Goals and Strategies. IPT has three phases: initial, intermediate, and final. During the initial phase, the connection between the patient's problem and interpersonal processes is explored by examining current and past relationships, and expectations about relationships and desired changes. In the intermediate phase, problem areas are the focus. Interpersonal disputes may be used to identify conflicts with others and alter expectations or faulty communication patterns to resolve the conflicts. Role transitions are dealt with by helping the patient accept the change or loss of a previous role and develop self-esteem through acquiring a sense of competence in the new role. Interpersonal skills are addressed by identifying social skills deficits, their link to social conflict, and their effect on relationships. During the final phase, termination and feelings of loss are discussed.

An Evaluation of Interpersonal Psychotherapy. IPT differs from psychodynamic therapy. While IPT involves recognition of intrapsychic conflicts, current problems are not interpreted as an expression of these conflicts. Current difficulties are attributed to current interpersonal problems. IPT also does not make the therapeutic relationship the primary focus of treatment (i.e., less reliance on transference). IPT is viewed by psychoanalytic therapists as supportive therapy that fails to resolve the underlying causes of emotional disorders. Controlled outcome studies have supported IPT, especially with unipolar depression.

Humanistic and Existential Psychotherapies

Humanistic and existential therapies are similar to psychoanalytic therapies in the core assumption that individuals must develop insight into their underlying needs and conflicts.

Carl Rogers's Person-Centered Therapy. Humanistic therapy was a reaction against Freudian and behavioral approaches and is based on the belief that people are innately good, and whose behavior is goal directed ad purposive. Self-actualization refers to the tendency toward personal growth to achieve personal fulfillment and unrealized potential. Psychoanalytic therapies assume that personality is determined by early childhood experiences, while humanistic therapists believe that people are free to shape their own futures. Psychodynamic therapists act as experts who make interpretations which give patients insight. Person-centered therapists encourage therapeutic relationships characterized by listening without interpretation and focusing on current experiences independently of childhood traumas. Psychoanalysts foster transference relationships while person-centered therapists reject techniques which place therapists in control. Rogers assumed that many techniques are unimportant, except to the extent that they encourage expression of three personal qualities of the therapist: 1) empathy (the ability to communicate to another person an understanding of what he/she is feeling and experiencing) occurs when the therapist immerses him/herself in the patient's world and perspective; 2) unconditional positive regard is the nonjudgmental acceptance of the patient's feelings and experiences, which conveys trust in the patient's own ability for self-understanding; and 3) genuineness is the therapist's ability to understand what another person is experiencing emotionally, which results from the therapist's complete trust of his/her own experience of the relationship with the patient. The major contribution of this therapy has been to improve understanding of how therapists aid the treatment process, and the role Rogers played in promoting empirical evaluation of psychotherapy. While research has failed to support the significance of empathy, unconditional positive regard, and genuineness as sufficient for effective treatment, they may aid improvement by facilitating the relationship.

Gestalt Therapy. Gestalt therapists also believe in the essentially positive nature of humans and their ability to make meaningful choices to improve themselves. However, they use a broader range of treatment techniques than person-centered therapists. Fritz Perls founded Gestalt therapy, which arose from an existential perspective. Problems are thought to arise when the individual's inborn positive potential cannot be freely expressed and developed. The therapy is founded on the principle that individuals need to integrate their experiences of self (thoughts and feelings) with their environmental circumstances; dichotomies between different aspects of functioning that interfere with personal growth and happiness need to be healed or integrated. Gestalt therapy focuses on the process of current experiences, with the goal of increasing awareness of feelings and external environments. Techniques to enhance awareness are based on immediate patient-therapist interactions. Therapists use frequent questioning of the patient's current feelings, emphasis on speaking directly to people, and encouragement of personal responsibility for feelings. The empty chair technique involves having the patient imagine that an individual is sitting in an empty chair while talking directly to the individual, and switching roles by sitting in the chair and talking from the other individual's perspective. Gestalt therapists have traditionally rejected quantitative research, and the available research focuses on process issues. There is some evidence that patient's ability to gain greater depths of experience during the empty chair technique were better able to resolve conflicts during sessions, and that the empty chair technique was more effective in reducing in-session psychological conflict than empathic reflection.

Behavior Therapy

Behavior therapy can be traced to three sources during the 1950s. First, Joseph Wolpe in South Africa developed and tested several treatment methods based on experimental research and principles of learning; he reported unprecedented rates of success with short-term psychotherapy. Second, Hans J. Eysenck in London defined behavior therapy as the application of learning principles and procedures to treatment of emotional disorders (an applied sciences which could be tested). Third, the principles of operant conditioning were applied to clinical problems in the United States. During the 1960s, behavior therapists had expanded their conceptualizations and methods to include classical and operant conditioning, developments in cognitive, social and developmental psychology, and Bandura's social learning theory. Today, there are three approaches to behavior therapy: 1) applied behavior analysis; 2) stimulus-response models; and 3) social learning theory.

Applied Behavior Analysis. This approach involves the application of the principles and procedures of operant conditioning to human problems and analyzes the effects of the environment on nature. This has been used most often with chronic mental patients in institutions, young children, and people who are mentally retarded, but is used with a wide range of other individuals as well.

The Stimulus-Response Approach. This approach involves the application of classical conditioning principles to clinical problems and emphasizes unobservable or mediational variables in explaining and modifying behavior. A mediational variable intervenes between an observable stimulus and response (i.e., anxiety). Systematic desensitization treatment is based on this approach.

Social Learning Theory. This approach depends on the theory that behavior is based on three separate but interacting regulatory systems: 1) external stimulus events (classical and operant conditioning); 2) external reinforcement; and 3) cognitive mediational processes (self-efficacy, self-regulation). Modeling is one of the best-known and most widely-used methods; behavior is learned or modified by systematically observing the behavior of a model. Clinical problems are thought to arise when a significant discrepancy develops between one's perceptions of events and objective reality. Efficacy expectations are people's feelings of confidence that they can cope with particular situations. Outcome expectations refer to people's beliefs that their actions will result in particular outcomes. Self-efficacy theory is a critical component of this approach. Attribution theory is also used to account for how one explains his/her attitudes and actions, and those of others.

Treatment Methods. The behavior therapist relies on empirical evidence about a technique's efficacy with a particular individual's problem, accepted clinical practice, intuitive skills and clinical experience to determine the most appropriate treatment method. Assertiveness and social skills training are two such methods. Assertion training involves having the therapist model appropriate assertive behavior, having the patient rehearse or role-play the behavior, having the therapist give feedback to the patient, and having the patient engage in assertive behavior in the real world. Patients are taught to avoid submissive and aggressive behaviors, while expressing their feelings honestly and directly. Communication principles (active listening, personal feedback, and self-disclosure and trust) is combined with instruction, modeling, and feedback of behavior rehearsal with this approach. Self-control strategies are used with both adults and children. Self-monitoring is used in assessment and treatment; the patient identifies and records specific thoughts, feelings and behaviors to become more aware of their specific problems. This method can also be used to help track the patient's improvement, to motivate change, and to facilitate self-motivation to engage in particular behaviors. Cognitive restructuring helps patients identify, challenge, and modify dysfunctional thoughts, and is often used in cognitive-behavioral therapy.

An Evaluation of Behavior Therapy. Advantages of this approach include its foundation on experimental psychology methods and principles, careful specification of treatment methods which can be evaluated in research, and the demonstrated efficacy of many of the methods in treating various clinical disorders. Criticisms of the approach center on the belief that treatment is superficial, focusing on symptoms while neglecting causes of the problems. Critics warn that symptom substitution (replacement of treated symptom with another because the underlying problem has not been resolved) may occur. However, behavior therapists also deal with causes of behavior; psychodynamic approaches and behavioral approaches differ on their views on the causes.

Cognitive Therapy

Rational Emotive Therapy. This approach, developed by Albert Ellis, assumes that individual's emotional disorders are rooted in irrational beliefs which are distortions of objective reality. These beliefs affect how individuals perceive experiences, which then lead to disorders. Therapy helps the patient identify irrational beliefs, replace them with more constructive, rational beliefs through cognitive rehearsal. The efficacy of RET has not been tested, partly because of the difficulty in specifying procedural components of treatment. Ellis has recently renamed his therapy rational emotive behavior therapy to more accurately reflect the comprehensive nature of the treatment.

Beck's Cognitive Therapy. This approach helps patients identify and modify dysfunctional thoughts and beliefs; negative thoughts and assumptions lead to negative moods, and a negative cycle can develop, which leads to clinical disorders. Patients keep written records, or dysfunctional thought records, to identify dysfunctional thoughts associated with emotional problems and which challenge the validity of those thoughts. Behavioral methods are used to correct dysfunctional thoughts by the therapist collaborating with the patient to test the assumptions. Figure 18.2 on page 589 and a transcript on pages 589-590 illustrate this process. This approach is clearly defined, which has facilitated empirical evaluation of its efficacy. Cognitive therapy has been demonstrated to be effective with depression and anxiety disorders.

Psychotherapy Integration

A 1990 poll of practicing psychotherapists demonstrated that about 1/3 used an eclectic approach to treatment, 1/3 used either a behavioral (18%) or a psychodynamic approach (15%), and the remaining used cognitive (10%), humanistic (7%) or systems (7%) approaches. Psychotherapy integration refers to the process of looking for commonalities among different and sometimes conflicting systems, learning from other perspectives, and integrating divergent methods.

Technical Eclecticism. This is a form of psychological treatment in which therapists draw on techniques from other systems of psychotherapy without necessarily subscribing to the theories behind the techniques. Lazarus, who founded this approach, has argued that there is insufficient development within the field to allow the integration of different concepts and techniques into a unified whole. Lazarus has developed this approach into multimodal therapy, which assesses patients across seven modalities represented by the acronym BASIC ID: behavior, affect, sensation, imagery, cognition, interpersonal behavior, and drugs (biology). This approach is illustrated in Table 18.1 on page 592 of the text.

The Common Factors Approach. Goldfried and Castonguay have supported this approach, which emphasizes clinical strategies common to all forms of psychological therapy, which vary from the highest level of abstraction (overall theoretical frameworks) to the lowest involving specific therapeutic techniques. Provision of new, corrective emotional experiences is an example of a common clinical strategy. The interpretation of which experiences are therapeutic, or why they are therapeutic, may differ across theoretic orientations. There are two distinct views of this approach: 1) there are more crucial commonalities that provide a foundation on which a more eclectic and integrated system of psychotherapy can be built; and 2) consensus on the types of strategies identified is limited to only the most superficial aspects of treatment, which assumes fundamentally different perspectives differ on basic issues which preclude integration.

The Effectiveness of Psychological Therapies

Eysenck argued in 1952 that there was no evidence that any psychotherapy was more effective than no treatment. Smith, Glass, and Miller (1980) argued that psychotherapy has many benefits. Arguments regarding the relative efficacy of various therapeutic approaches are even more controversial. Depending upon on the disorder, there is some evidence that one or more treatments are more effective than others. Another issue involves whether therapy has a deterioration effect, in which patients are worse after treatment. The term negative effect is used to describe the worsening of patient's problems as a result of therapy.

Meta-Analysis. This refers to a quantitative method of integrating the standardized results of a large number of separate studies. The effect size is a statistical index of treatment-produced change, which may be calculated by subtracting the mean of the control group from that of the treatment group, then dividing the difference by the standard deviation of the control group. Larger effect sizes indicate greater treatment effects. Proponents argue that meta-analysis is superior to qualitative reviews of literature because it minimizes subjectivity and bias. Critics argue against the practice of assigning equal weight to flawed and well-controlled studies, and have noted that subjective and arbitrary judgments are made about inclusion of studies, emphasis of methodological features, etc. Lastly, different meta-analyses have yielded inconsistent findings.

The Future of Psychotherapy

Health Care Reform. Psychotherapists have predicted that greater emphasis will be placed on present-centered, problem-focused, and time-limited psychological treatments in the future, and that psychodynamic approaches (which are among the most commonly used today) will be used much less often in the future. Government and private insurance programs will most likely reimburse patients only for time-limited treatments, and limit which kinds of therapy and which therapists can be used. The managed care movement is a system of health care in which all costs, options, and procedures are tightly controlled by health maintenance organizations (HMOs); the predicted shifts in reimbursement have been attributed to this movement. Increased emphasis on women's health care and on children's issues has also been predicted on the basis of the number of women going into the field of psychology. The Thinking About Gender Issues: The Feminization of Psychology box on page 569 explores this issue in more detail.

Psychotherapy and High Technology. Suicide and crisis hotlines have provided crisis intervention for many people, and therapists may take emergency phone calls from patients on occasion or maintain regular phone contact in between sessions. Networks of "telephone therapists" have been created as one form of electronic therapy (treatment delivered via telephone or computer, such as hotlines, phone networks, and electronic mail). This development has raised concerns about distinguishing between the type of problem which can adequately be handled by phone and those which cannot, the level of training appropriate for such services, and the possibilities for misuse. Virtual reality therapy, a computer-based means of manipulating the environment an individual experiences, has been used to treat patients with phobic disorders. This may be an effective means of achieving exposure to anxiety-provoking cues. Controlled studies must be conducted, however, to determine the efficacy of these methods.

KEY IDEAS AND OBJECTIVES FOR STUDENTS

After reading the chapter, you should be able to answer the following questions:

1. What are the characteristics of psychoanalytic therapies? What are the core concepts of this approach? How do ego-analytic and brief psychodynamic approaches differ from traditional Freudian psychoanalysis? What empirical is there for these approaches?

2. What are the characteristics and goals of interpersonal psychotherapy (IPT)? Is it effective?

3. What are the assumptions and characteristics of humanistic and existential therapies? What are the assumptions of Rogers' person-centered therapy, and of Gestalt therapy? What techniques are used with each?

4. What characterizes behavior therapy ? What has led to the use of the term cognitive-behavioral therapy (CBT) to describe the approach? What is the empirical evidence to support the efficacy and usefulness of behavior therapy techniques?

5. What are the assumptions of cognitive therapy, and how do the approaches of Ellis and Beck differ? Is there empirical support for these methods?

6. What is the goal of psychotherapy integration? What is technical eclecticism? What does the acronym BASIC ID represent?

7. Is there support for the effectiveness of psychological treatments? What is the controversy about this issue?

8. What are the predictions for the future of psychological treatment?

Sample Multiple-Choice Questions

1. Psychoanalysis originated with the work of
   a. Herman Rorschach
   b. Sigmund Freud
   c. Carl Jung
   d. Emil Kraeplin

2. Mary is in therapy with a psychologist who schedules individual sessions 4 times a week, every week. He has suggested that therapy will likely continue for several years. What type of psychotherapy is Mary's therapist probably using?
   a. Classical psychoanalysis
   b. Psychodynamic psychotherapy.
   c. Cognitive-behavioral psychotherapy.
   d. Family therapy.

3. Alesha was being seen by a therapist who focused on interpersonal roles and expectations. Alesha and her therapist discussed the roles that she plays and what would be lost if she were to change her roles. A great deal of attention was placed on the development of interpersonal skills and social difficulties. Alesha's therapist was likely using methods derived from ___________________.
   a. psychodynamic psychotherapy.
   b. social learning theory.
   c. ego-analytic theory.
   d. interpersonal psychotherapy.

4. Humanistic theory focuses on ___________________ as a major source of human motivation.
   a. self-actualization
   b. the unconscious
   c. environmental reinforcement
   d the id

5. Research by Rogers and his colleagues identified 3 characteristics of therapists that today are encouraged by all therapy approaches. Which of the following is <u>not</u> one of the three personal qualities of therapists?
   a. Attractiveness
   b. Empathy
   c. Genuineness
   d. Unconditional Positive Regard

6. Myron wants to work with chronic institutionalized mental patients. He talks with his undergraduate advisor about career opportunities and decides to apply to a clinical psychology program. What should Myron look for in selecting a graduate program? The program should offer training in
   a. applied behavior analysis
   b. psychoanalysis
   c. social learning theory
   d. person-centered psychotherapy

7. Cognitive restructuring is designed to help patients identify and modify ____________________.
   a. dysfunctional thinking patterns.
   b. social relationships.
   c. depressive symptoms.
   d. overt patterns of behavior.

8. Kikki sought treatment for depression at a medical school near her home town. The Mood Disorders Clinic used a cognitive therapy program. Which of the following assessment strategies will the staff likely give Kikki to assess her depression?
   a. MMPI
   b. Rorschach Test.
   c. Beck Depression Inventory
   d. Schedule of Recent Events.

9 The type of therapy most often linked to technical eclecticism is ____________________.
   a. multimodal therapy
   b. cognitive-behavioral therapy
   c. brief psychodynamic psychotherapy
   d. interpersonal psychotherapy

10. The majority of all graduates from clinical psychology programs are ________.
   a. men
   b. women
   c. evenly split between men and women
   d. men, but signs are present that more women than ever are enrolling in these programs.

Answer Key

1. b
2. a
3. d
4. a
5. a
6. a
7. a
8. c
9. a
10. b

CHAPTER 19 MARITAL, FAMILY, GROUP AND COMMUNITY THERAPIES

Marital Therapy

Prevalence and Impact of Marital Problems

Divorce and marital separation rank second and third, respectively, as the most significant life stressors, exceeded only by the death of a spouse. At least half of depressed women seeking treatment have clinically significant marital problems, and most couples with sexual problems or couples in which one spouse has alcohol or drug dependency problems have significant marital problems as well. In some cases marital problems may be a consequence of other problems such as schizophrenia.

Divorce and separation have widespread consequences. The high rates of depression and suicide among adolescents and young adults, and depression have been attributed to the increase is the rise in divorce. Marital problems are also associated with decreases in biological functioning. Both divorce and marital disruption appear to lead to decreases in immune function; however, it is not clear that reductions in immune function associated with marital problems influence the likelihood of developing infections or other diseases. But many clinicians presume that the likelihood of infections and diseases does increase if the stressors are intense and occur over a long period. Even more striking are the data showing that married men and women have lower risks of dying than those who are not married.

Treatment of Marital/Relationship Problems

Marital therapy aims to help couples improve their communication, develop insight into their problems, and explore feelings. Therapies can be used with unmarried couples, gay or lesbian couples, elderly couples, or with couples who wish to separate and divorce on amicable terms (e.g., to minimize the negative impact on the children). Conjoint sessions in which both partners are present are usually conducted when both partners are willing to attend therapy.

Couples who profit most from therapy have some commitment to remain together and some love or caring for each other. In assessment sessions, over 50 percent of men and women report that their main problem is communication. About one-third of men and women report decreased interest in sexual interactions and conflicting personality styles, and about 10% report lack of affection and love.

Changing Patterns of Communication. Regardless of theoretical orientation, most marital therapies attempt to analyze and change communication patterns by getting each partner to listen to the other with concern and understanding. To develop mutual understanding, the therapist helps each partner express empathy for the other's feelings and needs. Once they understand and empathize with each other, the couple can begin to resolve differences and find ways to satisfy each other's needs. Couples are encouraged to communicate directly and in a constructive way, avoiding criticism in favor of specific requests and suggestions. Once communication improves, therapy often turns to problem-solving skills. Partners are encouraged to define a problem, brainstorm possible solutions, and choose a solution.

<u>Changing Attitudes</u>. Many distressed husbands and wives have irrational attitudes and/or unrealistic expectations of their partners and of marriage. These include unrealistic expectations that spouses/partners should always agree with each other if they love each other, that marriage should satisfy all one's needs, and attributing the partner's negative behaviors to stable traits.

<u>Changing Behavior</u>. Increasing positive behaviors may be accomplished by love days or caring days in which each person agrees to engage in specific behaviors that please his/her partner. This may prompt positive actions and interactions and demonstrate that both partners are willing to improve the marriage.

Effectiveness of Marital Therapy

If increasing marital satisfaction is the goal, then insight-oriented therapies focusing on unconscious factors that influence choice of mate and later marital conflicts are not effective. On the other hand, if insight concerns the kinds of behaviors that should be changed to make the marriage better, marital satisfaction increases. A comparison of insight-oriented marital therapy and behavioral marital therapy indicated that the insight-oriented marital therapy fared much better at follow-up. Prior to treatment, most couples are extremely dissatisfied; after treatment, clients are more satisfied with their relationships but they are still slightly dissatisfying. Between 60-90% of couples stay married several years after treatment. In some cases, however, divorce may be a more desirable outcome (e.g., physically abusive relationships).

Family Therapy

Family Systems Therapy

This is the most common approach to treating families and treats the family as a dynamic system in which each member's role affect each other member and the system as a whole. Relationships among family members are emphasized more than the specific difficulties of an individual family member. Boundaries which normally separate parents and children may become blurred when two family members from different generations form a tight bond and exclude another member. Alternatively, a strained relationship between two members may be avoided by focusing on a third member (child) as a target of criticism, or by making the person a scapegoat. Therapy utilizes a number of specific techniques.

<u>Reframing</u>. Reframing means conceptualizing a problem in a new way. Family members are asked to frame the presenting problem in a new light by viewing an individual's problem as a family problem and removing blame from the person seen as causing or having the problem. This lessens the negative views or attributions about the person identified as "the problem."

<u>Validation</u>. Validation refers to the expressing understanding of individual family members' feelings and desires. This occurs prior to making changes in family dynamics.

Paradoxical Directives. The therapist encourages the client to do something that seems contradictory, such as prescribing the actual symptom the client wishes to eliminate. This may act to remove the patient's need to have the problem, and this technique works well with resistant teenagers and young adults.

Family therapy approaches have not been as rigorously evaluated. However, they have proven useful in treating drug abuse problems, anorexia, and bulimia. Structural family therapy is a treatment approach in which the family is viewed as the unit to change by altering the entire family system by assessing and restructuring the roles and relationships between the various family members. This approach is often used with drug abuse. Some research has shown that 65-76% of clients show improvement, but they were not well-controlled. There is tentative support for the effectiveness of family therapy, however.

Problem-Solving Therapy

The second major treatment approach directed at changing families is problem-solving therapy, which has somewhat more focused goals than family systems therapy. Although both approaches view the family as the unit to change, changes in communication or behavior for a dyad (such as father/son) or an individual (for instance a child or teenager) are acceptable goals for problem-solving treatments. Problem-solving approaches consist of four basic phases: 1) defining the problem; 2) generating alternative solutions to the defined problem before family members criticize solutions (sometimes called brainstorming); 3) evaluating the alternative solutions; and 4) implementing the best available solutions. This approach has been effective with depressed and schizophrenic individuals' families.

Integration of Family and Behavior Therapy

Sometimes behavior therapy strategies can be more effective when combined with family therapies. Alexander and Parsons developed a systems-behavioral approach for families of delinquent families. This blends behavioral and family systems perspectives with an emphasis on parental disciplinary strategies. Combining behavioral parent-training and family systems approaches was more effective in treating families for child abuse and neglect than either approach alone. Combined approaches have also been found to be effective with populations that are hard to reach and difficult to treat (e.g., inner-city families, aggressive and delinquent children).

Group Therapy

Group therapy consists of meetings of a small group of individuals to obtain and provide mutual support and guidance in coping with psychological problems. Group approaches are employed for almost every psychological problem, and one survey found that more Americans participate in some form of group therapy than in any other type of therapy. This popularity may be due to the lower cost compared to individual treatment, and the fact that group approaches help individuals with problems that are very difficult to treat individually, such as alcoholism. More pressure to change behavior may be made by a group and groups can offer the comfort of being with others dealing with the same problems.

Gestalt Therapy

Gestalt therapy is a humanistically oriented therapy in which participants are encouraged to complete "unfinished business" by examining the past for unresolved conflicts while dealing with current life issues and making the most of each day. Little research evaluating gestalt therapy exists; however, many have testified to its value. Gestalt therapy has been shown to be effective in some areas (e.g., marital therapy or marital enrichment) and has promising initial results in others (e.g. decision making and depression).

Alcoholics Anonymous

Alcoholics Anonymous (AA) was founded in 1935 by Dr. Bob and Bill W as a volunteer self-help organization to help individuals maintain sobriety. AA relies on a "buddy" or a sponsor who has been able to remain sober for some time to provide support and encouragement to a new member trying to stop drinking. A 12-step program is the basis for this approach, which focuses on problem-focused discussions about how to resist drinking and an admission that members cannot control themselves if they use alcohol. There are four critical treatment ingredients: 1) it offers a substitute for drinking at the bars, because AA meetings are held at hours that compete with those of bars; 2) AA makes it clear that the alcoholic cannot drink without becoming dependent; 3) it teaches the individual how to cope with feelings of loneliness; and 4) it offers role models, in the form of sober people who have successfully coped with their desire to have a drink.

AA's effects are very difficult to ascertain, even though it has been a major force in treating alcoholism for over 50 years. Few controlled evaluations exist; this research shows that between 25 to 50 percent of individuals who remain in the program are sober after one year. Whatever the overall effectiveness of AA, however, millions of people clearly find it helpful.

Community Therapy

Therapeutic Communities

The Therapeutic community grew out of dissatisfaction with the limitations of traditional hospital treatments for mentally ill patients. This approach involves patients in an institutional setting who are treated as normally as possible by living in a family-style environment and being encouraged to develop routines and participate in chores. They generally revolve around regular meetings in a homelike atmosphere. This approach became a model for many halfway houses, which are facilities for individuals released from a hospital or other treatment program who need more supervision and monitoring than their homes and families can provide. With adequate community follow-up, these approaches can be effective in facilitating return to the community. Compared to standard hospital after-care, halfway houses for mental patients result in less frequent readmittance to mental hospitals and more employment.

Community Psychology

Therapeutic communities focus primarily on changing problematic behavior or conditions. In contrast, community psychology, developed in the 1960s and 1970s, attempts to prevent problems and to teach new skills. Community programs have involved television programs and commercials to foster health-promoting behaviors (e.g., exercising, smoking cessation), and various numbers of people from small groups to entire communities. Prevention has always been a major focus of community psychology, with three basic types of programs. Primary prevention programs attempt to prevent the development of new problems in a population, mainly through education. Secondary prevention programs attempt to detect problems early on in order to prevent their further escalation. Tertiary prevention aims to reduce long-term consequences of a problem.

KEY IDEAS AND OBJECTIVES FOR STUDENTS

After reading the chapter, you should be able to answer each of the following questions:

1. How stressful are divorce and marital separation? What is the relationship between depression in women and marital problems?

2. What are the goals and emphasis of marital therapy? With whom is it used? What types of approaches are used in marital therapy?

3. What are the characteristics and goals of family systems therapy? What are the characteristics and goals of problem-solving therapy?

4. What are the characteristics of group therapy? What are the characteristics of Gestalt group therapy?

5. What are the characteristics of Alcoholics Anonymous (AA)?

6. What approaches are used in therapeutic communities?

Marital, Family, Group and Community Therapies in the Movies

Kramer vs Kramer (1979, Columbia Tri-Star, 105 min). This movie could be shown to illustrate the issues relevant to marital discord and divorce, as well as family systems issues. The central characters in this film are a young couple (played by Meryl Streep and Dustin Hoffman) and their young son. When the wife leaves, the husband must assume primary caretaking of his son. Family dynamics clearly change when this occurs. When the wife returns and the couple agree to divorce, a custody dispute ensues. The stress this produces for the young child is clearly portrayed. This film could be used to help students consider the research on marital discord and divorce, as well as on different therapy approaches which may have prevented the divorce in this family.

Questions after watching the movie:

1. Given the text's summary of the characteristics of couples seeking marital therapy, how well did the movie do in presenting an accurate portrayal of a couple with significant discord? What "errors" (including errors of omission and commission) were made?

2. What were the family dynamics prior to separation, immediately following separation, and during the custody dispute? How well did the characters' behaviors fit with the family systems model?

3. What treatments do you think might have been appropriate prior to the couple separating? How successful do you think treatment would have been?

4. If you were to be a consultant on a "remake" of this film, what advice would you give the director to help make the relationships issues more contemporary?

Sample Multiple-Choice Questions

1. Most couples who are experiencing marital difficulties rank _______________ as their most important problem.
   a. money
   b. communication
   c. love
   d. sex

2. At least ___________ of the depressed women who seek treatment have clinically significant marital difficulties.
   a. 10%
   b. 25%
   c. 50%
   d. 65%

3. Which of the following problems are more likely to reported by women than men at the initial marital assessment?
   a. personality styles
   b. affect/love
   c. physical aggression
   d. all of the above.

4. Brett and Tammy arrive at a marriage therapy clinic for an initial interview. The therapist starts by saying that she wants to meet individually with each of them as part of the general assessment. Is this common or has the therapist learned something about the couple that she is trying to explore.
   a. Yes, this is common.
   b. No, this is uncommon and likely means that she suspects spousal abuse.
   c. No, this is uncommon and likely means that she suspects that Brett has an alcohol problem.
   d. No, this is uncommon and likely means that she suspects infidelity.

5. Margarita met with Dr. Carey about her problems at home. Margarita reports feeling tense and irritable and has difficulty communicating with her husband or her children. Her mother lives in the home and suggested that Margarita needed to see a therapist to learn to be a better wife. Dr. Carey shared that he felt that Margarita was merely the person her family identified as having a problem, and that each member of the family probably plays a role. He suggested that therapy should involve the whole family: herself, her husband, her children and her mother. What is Dr. Carey's theoretical approach to psychotherapy?
   a. Social Learning
   b. Psychodynamic
   c. Family Systems
   d. Interpersonal

6. ____________________ is a characteristic found both in Mexican American families and in families with origins in Puerto Rico that helps maintain traditional values..
   a. Familism
   b. Egalitarian
   c. Paternalism
   d. Maternalism

7. A treatment approach in which a small group of individuals meet to obtain mutual support and guidance in coping with psychological problems is called _______________.
   a. structural family therapy
   b. conjoint therapy
   c. group therapy
   d. gestalt therapy

8. The most successful AA members regularly attend meetings. According to an AA survey, how often do "regularly attending" member attend?
   a. One meeting a month
   b. Two meetings a month
   c. One meeting a week
   d. Four meetings a week

9. Prevention of new problems in a population is ____________ prevention.
   a. primary
   b. secondary
   c. tertiary
   d. community

10. The detection of problems early on in order to reduce their intensity and prevent further escalation is ______________ prevention.
    a. primary
    b. secondary
    c. tertiary
    d. community

Answer Key

1. b
2. c
3. a
4. a
5. c
6. a
7. c
8. d
9. a
10. b

CHAPTER 20 BIOLOGICAL THERAPIES

Medications

Three major classes of biological treatments are presented: medication (i.e., antidepressants, lithium, antianxiety medication, antipsychotic medication, and psychostimulants); electroconvulsive therapy (ECT); and psychosurgery. Pychotropic medications are drugs used to change feelings, thoughts, and behavior.

Antidepressants. The medications used to treat depression can be grouped into three classes: selective serotonin re-uptake inhibitors (SSRIs), tricyclic antidepressants (TCAs), and monoamine oxidase inhibitors (MAOIs). Selective serotonin re-uptake inhibitors (SSRIs) are called "selective" because they are said to affect serotonergic systems with very little effect on other neurotransmitter systems. Two new SSRI medications, Zoloft and Paxil, are classified as SSRIs, along with Prozac. Although the exact biochemical causes of depression are not clearly known, it is believed that serotonin and norepinephrine are depleted in depressed individuals. Some experts believe that Prozac makes more serotonin available by blocking its reuptake or reabsorption of serotonin. Some clinicians believe that among SSRIs, Prozac has the fewest side effects; it has the added advantage of being able to be given at the same dosage over the entire course of treatment. Even so, Prozac produces insomnia, nervousness, restlessness, and anxiety in some individuals.

Tricylic antidepressants have a three-ring molecular structure. Researchers believe that tricyclics interfere with or block the re-uptake of norepinephrine and serotonin at the nerve cell after it has fired. However, tricyclic antidepressants clearly have a positive mood elevating effect on many depressed individuals. Initial effects on sleep and appetite usually occur after one or two weeks of treatment. However, antidepressant effects may not be achieved until the third or fourth week, and a complete trial should last six weeks. The most common side effects of high doses of tricyclics are dry mouth, fatigue, constipation, difficulty in urination, memory difficulty, dizziness, and weight gain. Optimal duration of treatment is four to six months for an acute episode of depression, with gradual withdrawal of medication advised three to five months after the initial antidepressant effects of the medication are observed.

Combined effects of antidepressant medication and psychotherapy are often seen as the most effective way to treat depression. Persons with severe or chronic depression who are partial responders to either treatment alone (psychotherapy or medication) may benefit from combining psychological and pharmacological treatments. However, evidence is not consistent about the value of combining medication and psychotherapy, and where combined effects are superior, patients are severely depressed.

MAO inhibitors are medications that block the action of MAO (monoamine oxidase), and are the third major type of medication used to treat depression. Because of the negative side effects of MAO inhibitors, they are used primarily when a patient does not respond to other antidepressant medications. The MAO inhibitors prevent the breakdown of the neurotransmitters, norepinephrine and serotonin, thereby keeping more of these substances available for uptake. In turn, their availability reduces depression. When MAO inhibitors are taken with foods high in tyramine, such as yeast, chocolate, beer, and various wines, serious physical reactions occur such as severe headaches, heart palpitations, stroke or even death. These side effects occur because tyramine is absorbed rapidly in combination with the MAO medication, in turn leading to a life-threatening increase in blood pressure. Therefore, patients taking MAO inhibitors cannot eat even small amounts of certain foods. Because of the toxicity and potential lethal effects of the MAO inhibitors, they are generally used with individuals who do not respond to other available medications.

Other antidepressants include Wellbutrin and Desyrel. Neither is included among the three classes of medications discussed earlier. Wellbutrin is sometimes used as an alternative to Prozac for patients who experience sexual problems. Unfortunately, Wellbutrin sometimes produces seizures. Desyrel does not block serotonin. Its mechanism of antidepressant action is unclear. Desyrel is sometimes is used in combination with Prozac to counter the insomnia that Prozac sometimes produces. Desyrel has a sedative quality that makes it effective at night in helping patients sleep. However, clinicians have repeatedly noted that Desyrel seems less effective than other antidepressants in treating severe depression and it has a very painful though rare side effect, namely a constant erection.

Secondary clinical uses of antidepressant medication include the treatment of panic disorder with agoraphobia, obsessive-compulsive disorders, bulimia nervosa, and aggressive-impulsive behavior. The tricyclic antidepressant, Anafranil, has reduced the symptoms of obsessive-compulsive children and adults. The SSRI, Prozac, has also led to significant reductions in obsessions and compulsions. Antidepressants are also used to treat eating disorders such as bulimia nervosa.

Lithium. This medication is frequently prescribed to treat patients suffering from manic episodes of bipolar disorder because it normalizes moods. It is clearly the treatment of choice for manic-depressives, effective in approximately 60-70 percent of cases. Lithium prevents the characteristic swings from extreme highs to extreme lows. Lithium has a small " therapeutic window" or dose level that is therapeutic rather than toxic. At least six possible mechanisms have been hypothesized to account for Lithium's effects, but alterations in brain levels of serotonin and norepinephrine are prominent among these views.

Antianxiety Medications. Many of the early antianxiety medications, such as chloral hydrate, were addictive and could not be used for prolonged periods of time. Benzodiazepines are the most commonly used class of antianxiety medications used today. This includes Valium, Xanax, and Halcion. All members of this class of medications are equally effective in treating anxiety. The eight most frequently prescribed benzodiazepines are presented in Table 20.3 on page 633. Many call the benzodiazepines by a more technical name, anxiolytics, literally meaning "anxiety looseners". A positive effect of these drugs is their calming effects. Approximately 65-70% of individuals report these effects, usually within the first week. Negative effects include drowsiness and lack of coordination, and dangerous interactions with alcohol. Tolerance and withdrawal symptoms that appear on abrupt termination of use are additional problems with these medications. Benzodiazepines generally inhibit the central nervous system by acting on specific receptor sites that affect neurotransmitters in the brain, leading to reduced nerve cell firing. Relief from anxiety is almost directly proportional to the dosage taken; as tolerance develops, the dosage must be increased to obtain the same level of anxiety reduction. Physiological and psychological dependency on the benzodiazepines may develop from this increased tolerance. Withdrawal should occur gradually, not all at once, to minimize anxiety, irritability, sleep disturbance, and impaired memory.

Buspirone (BuSpar) is an antianxiety medication that is chemically unrelated to the benzodiazepines, and its mechanisms of action are unknown. It does not have the potential for addiction of the benzodiazepines, and does not have significant sedating effects nor the risk of dependence. It does not impair coordination. However, BuSpar does have some negative side effects, however, such as dizziness, faintness, and mild drowsiness. Finally, BuSpar is generally not useful for individuals who did not respond to the benzodiazepines.

Antipsychotic Medications. These medications are sometimes called major tranquilizers, because one of their most common side effects is sedation. They are also called neuroleptics because they have side effects that influence the neurological system. French surgeon Henri Laborit observed that patients given medication to reduce blood pressure were markedly less anxious. In 1952, French psychiatrists Jean Delay and Pierre Deniker gave Thorazine (a variation of the medication used by surgeon Laborit) to a variety of psychiatric patients; many showed reductions in anxiety and a marked decrease of hallucinations and delusions. Positive effects include the ability of schizophrenic patients (who had been hospitalized for years) to return to their jobs and families (see Chapter 13, Schizophrenia). This contributed to the deinstitutionalization trend that began in the 1960s. The positive effects of antipsychotic medications occur in about 80-90 percent of schizophrenics. Negative effects include muscle rigidity, stooped posture, unusual shuffling gate, and even occasional drooling. These effects are similar to the symptoms of Parkinson's disease, and are called Parkinsonian effects. Another related negative side effect is tardive dyskinesia, characterized by slowed movements of the face, tongue, and neck muscles. For many patients, such motor abnormalities are irreversible; for others, there is a reduction in symptoms once medication is discontinued.

The serious side effects of many antipsychotic medications and the fact that some individuals are not responsive to antipsychotic medications has led researchers to search for alternatives. Clozaril appears useful for some of the 10-20% of schizophrenics unresponsive to generally available antipsychotic medications. Clozaril does not have significant negative effects on motor functioning; however, it causes diminished white blood cell count in some patients which requires careful and costly monitoring. Risperdal (risperidone) inhibits both dopamine and serotonin, and reduces both positive and negative symptoms of schizophrenia. Because it has a low incidence of tardive dyskinesia, Risperdal is increasingly becoming one of the first choice medications in treating schizophrenic patients. Combined use of antipsychotic medication and family therapy may be used when families are available and supportive. This may result in fewer hospitalizations for many schizophrenic patients.

Psychostimulants. Psychostimulants are used primarily to increase attention span and decrease restlessness in children. In addition, physicians prescribe psychostimulants for a sleeping disorder, narcolepsy. Research by psychologist Keith Conners showed that hyperactive children with attentional problems showed a positive response to psychostimulant medication. The three most commonly used psychostimulant medications are Ritalin (methylphenidate), Dexedrine (dextroamphetamine), and Cylert (magnesium pemoline). Although they are generally equally effective, Ritalin is used most often with children. Positive effects include increased attention and decreased restlessness, and improved fine motor skills performance. Negative effects include increased heart rate, blood pressure, and central nervous system responsivity. In adults, marked feelings of euphoria, and increased energy levels may occur. It is now clear that they are addictive and dangerous for adults. However, when administered appropriately, psychostimulants are not addictive to children.

Combined psychostimulants and other therapy are often used, because increases in academic performance as reflected on standard achievement tests have not been associated with taking psychostimulant medication. Professionals believe that hyperactive children's critical problems in learning new academic and social skills cannot be addressed simply with medication. A combined approach using medication and behavior therapy or family therapy intervention may be the treatment of choice for some.

Secondary clinical uses of psychostimulants include treatment of a sleep disorder called narcolepsy. Narcolepsy is a rare sleep disorder in which a person falls asleep suddenly at inappropriate times and places. Psychostimulants often decrease the frequency of narcoleptic sleep attacks and drowsiness. Another use of psychostimulants is with people who are depressed and do not respond to antidepressants.

Electroconvulsive Therapy (ECT)

Discovery. Electroshock treatment is the use of an electrical current through the brain to produce a brief convulsion. ECT became an accepted treatment choice for schizophrenia in the 1940s to 1960s, and was used with other disorders, such as severe depression. Concern was raised over bone fractures, memory loss, and heart complications following ECT, and the use of ECT to control violent and aggressive patients. Research in the 1960s and 1970s led to safer and more effective ECT treatment. Brief electrical impulses were used at lower voltages than in earlier decades. In addition, placing electrodes on only one side of the head resulted in fewer side effects than when electrodes were used on both sides. Memory loss is then usually only temporary. ECT remains a generally safe, rapid and effective treatment for depression.

Current Use. Patients undergoing ECT receive a light, general anesthesia to make them sleep prior to treatment, and are injected with a muscle relaxant to prevent violent muscle contractions. Seizures are then induced by passing 150 volts of electricity through electrodes just above the temple. The seizure lasts approximately one minute and the patient awakens within 5 to 10 minutes. Today, ECT is most commonly used in treating patients with severe, long-lasting depression who have not responded to or cannot tolerate the side effects of various antidepressant medications, often these are elderly patients.

Psychosurgery

Psychosurgery is the most controversial treatment, and involves the selective surgical removal of part of the brain or the destruction of nerve pathways to influence behavior. It was developed before the discovery of effective antipsychotic medications at a time when no effective treatments existed for many psychiatric disorders. The earliest psychosurgeries removed the frontal lobes (prefrontal lobotomy) from schizophrenic patients. As a result, many patients became apathetic and inactive, and over half became mute. Today, very limited forms of psychosurgery are performed on patients with specific severe and intractable disorders. It is largely confined to the treatment of severely obsessive-compulsive individuals or to patients with incapacitating depression associated with severe anxiety. Treatment remains controversial in treating obsessive-compulsive behavior. Nonetheless, the treatment holds hope for some patients whose lives have been severely handicapped by obsessions and compulsions.

KEY IDEAS AND OBJECTIVES FOR STUDENTS

After reading the chapter, you should be able to answer each of the following questions:

1. What are the primary classes of antidepressants?

2. How effective is Prozac, and what are its side effects? How do tricyclic antidepressants appear to elevate mood? What are the side effects of MAO inhibitors?

3. What drugs are used in treating bipolar disorder? Which is most effective?

4. How effective are the benzodiazepines? What are their positive effects? What are their negative effects?

5. How effective is Buspirone (BuSpar) and for whom is it used? What are its advantages over other antianxiety medications?

6. What are the positive effects of antipsychotic medications? What are their side effects?

7. What are the new antipsychotic medications, and what are the advantages and disadvantages of these drugs?

8. What are the positive and negative effects of psychostimulant medication for children with attention-deficit/hyperactivity disorder? How do they affect adults? Are they effective in the treatment of narcolepsy?

9. What are the characteristics of electroconvulsive or electroshock therapy as it used today? How does this differ from its use in the past? For whom and under what conditions is this treatment effective?

10. How is psychosurgery used today? Is it effective?

Biological Therapies in the Movies

One Flew Over the Cuckoo's Nest (1975, Republic Pictures Home Video, 133 min). This film provides a perspective from the view of a patient confined to a mental hospital for evaluation. The patient (played by Jack Nicholson) is given ECT and, eventually, psychosurgery (probably a frontal lobotomy). The film provides a reasonable demonstration of the way in which ECT was initially used and raises issues concerning its misuse as a means of punishing or controlling patients. The consequences of psychosurgery are portrayed as very severe. These scenes from the film could be used to consider the controversy surrounding these two treatments, and the ways in which they are typically used today.

Questions after watching the movie:

1. Given the text's description of the way in which ECT was used prior to the 1970s, how well did the movie portray this method of treatment? What "errors" (including errors of omission and commission) did the movie make in terms of the consequences of ECT?

2. How did the ECT portrayed in the film differ from the way in which ECT is used today? What were the major similarities and differences?

3. What were the effects of the psychosurgery on the patient's functioning? How did his behavior, emotional expressiveness, and activity level change after the surgery? How accurate was the movie in portraying the consequences of psychosurgery?

4. If you were to be a consultant on a "remake" of this film, what advice would you give the director to help you make the treatments more contemporary?

Sample Multiple-Choice Questions

1. Antidepressants can be grouped into three classes. Which of the following is NOT one of these classes?
   a. anxiolytic selectives
   b. selective serotonin reuptake inhibitors
   c. tricyclic antidepressants
   d. monoamine oxidase inhibitors

2. While the exact cause of depression is unknown, levels of ________ appear to be depleted in depressed individuals.
   a. serotonin
   b. norepinephrine
   c. serotonin and norepinephrine
   d. none of the above

3. Which of the following statements about Lithium is TRUE?

   a. Lithium is effective for only 20 to 30 percent of patients with manic-depressive or bipolar disorder.
   b. Lithium is very effective in treating major depression and is usually the only drug given during depressive episodes.
   c. Lithium normalizes depressed mood, but has little effect on manic episodes.
   d. Lithium has a small "therapeutic window," meaning that the dose that is effective is very close to the dose that is toxic.

4. The early antianxiety drugs were problematic because _______.
   a. they were addictive
   b. they were only effective for women
   c. they were only effective for men
   d. they caused severe insomnia

5. Larry is 67 years old and is an alcoholic. He has been experiencing a great deal of anxiety and worry because his wife had a heart attack. His physician, Dr. Weston, decides to prescribe an antianxiety medication. She is most likely to prescribe _______.
   a. Valium
   b. Prozac
   c. BuSpar
   d. Halcion

6. Deinstitutionalization, in which hospitals markedly reduced the number of patients in hospitals by returning them to the community, was the result of the discovery of ________ drugs.
   a. antidepressant
   b. antianxiety
   c. antipsychotic
   d. psychostimulant

7. The new antipsychotic medication which does not have significant negative effects on motor functioning, which is useful for those individuals who are unresponsive to common antipsychotic medication, but which can result in lowered white blood cell count, is ________.
   a. Thorazine, or chlorpromazine
   b. Haldol, or haloperidol
   c. Clozaril, or clozapine
   d. Mellaril, or thioridazine

8. Jermaine is a ten-year-old boy who has been diagnosed with attention-deficit/hyperactivity disorder. He has trouble remaining seated, paying attention, and completing assignments in his classroom. His teacher notices a significant improvement in his behavior and tells his parents that he is completing his assignment, staying in his seat, and that his handwriting has improved. Jermaine's parents tell his teacher that he started taking medication for his AD/HD. What medication is Jermaine most likely taking?
   a. Prozac
   b. Ritalin
   c. Haldol
   d. Tegretol

9. Electroshock treatment has been found to ________.
   a. cause structural brain damage in approximately 20 percent of patients
   b. cause increased thoughts of suicide in approximately 50 percent of patients
   c. be acceptable to approximately 80 percent of patients treated with ECT
   d. be ineffective in reducing depression for severely depressed individuals

10. Margaret has been plagued by severe obsessive-compulsive disorder for most of her adult life. She is unable to work and her previous treatment with cognitive-behavior therapy. Medication with antidepressants and antianxiety drugs has also been unsuccessful. Her physician has consulted with experts and has concluded that ________ is likely to be effective in reducing her obsessions and compulsions.
    a. electroshock treatment
    b. psychostimulant medication
    c. psychosurgery
    d. antipsychotic medication

Answer Key

1. a
2. c
3. d
4. a
5. c
6. c
7. c
8. b
9. c
10. c

CHAPTER 21 LEGAL AND ETHICAL ISSUES

Legal issues concern the rights and freedoms that all persons, including those who are mentally or medically impaired, can expect from society and what society in turn can expect from them. Some of the issues are quite old and date back to antiquity. Other issues are more specific to the age and place we live in today.

Mental Health Professionals and the Law

Mental health professionals are routinely called as expert witnesses during court proceedings. They help answer such difficult questions as whether a defendant is competent to stand trial, is dangerous and should be involuntarily committed for psychiatric treatment, or was psychologically incapacitated when the crime he or she is accused of was committed. Although the ultimate decision is made by a judge, psychologists and psychiatrists are often asked their opinions as experts on behavior before decisions are made.

Nearly everyone agrees that these professionals have important roles to play; the quality of these professional judgments has been disappointing for several reasons.

First, mental health professionals who serve as expert witnesses are typically asked to answer some of the hardest human questions imaginable. They may be asked to predict the likelihood that a person will be dangerous to society or to herself in the future or to decide which parent will provide the best care for a child.

Second, the adversarial nature of the US legal system requires each side in a civil or criminal matter to try to convince a judge that their viewpoint is correct. In cases in which a judgment call must be relied on, both sides can usually find a mental health professional willing to support its contention.

Third, a great deal of training and experience is required to become a competent expert witness. Research on training expert witnesses suggest that psychologists are best at three things: (a) detecting <u>malingering</u> (faking an illness or disorder); (b) predicting violent behavior, especially on a short-term basis; and (c) evaluating competency to stand trial. However, specialized training is needed in order to do these things effectively.

Dangerousness and the Duty to Warn

Judgments about <u>dangerousness</u> are among the most frequently sought, important, and difficult of those mental health professionals are asked to make. They are difficult since the professional is not often given all the information necessary to make a sure call and decisions must be made quickly. The primary reason that it is difficult to predict long-term dangerousness is that the likelihood of violent acts seems to depend more on the immediate circumstances preceding the violence than on the attacker's personality. Recently, however, four kinds of risk factors for violence have been identified: (a) anger control capacity and the ability to meet threats without violence, (b) arrests and conviction history and history of diligence in keeping psychiatric treatment appointments, (c) living arrangements and family situation, and (d) delusions, hallucinations, and fantasies of violence.

Despite the difficulty of predicting dangerousness over the long term, since 1974, there has been a legal responsibility of psychotherapists to warn persons threatened during the course of psychotherapy. The decision is known as the Tarrasoff standard. In this court decision, it was specified that only therapists have the clear duty to warn, presumably on the assumption that they know their patients better can thus make the difficult judgment of dangerousness more accurately than anyone else. States vary in the extent with which therapists responsible to warn or protect and professional organizations have begun to develop standards that help therapists limit their Tarasoff liability.

Although clinicians are more confident that they can accurately predict the seriousness of a suicide threat or attempt, data supporting this conviction are not very convincing. Nonetheless, psychologists and psychiatrists have developed criteria for making this judgment.

Civil Commitment

When hospitalization is clearly indicated but the patient refuses to comply, civil commitment (or involuntary hospitalization) may be necessary. Several factors influence this decision. First, one must predict the level of dangerousness (to self and others). The Index of Dangerousness Indicators (TRIAD) has been developed to allow for more reliable and valid measure of dangerousness. Second, individuals who do not meet the dangerousness criterion but clearly do require and would benefit from treatment can be committed if they cannot exercise the good judgment required to know they are sick, incapacitated, and in need of treatment. These individuals are said to have a grave disability. Third, in most states, plans for civil commitment must involve a least restrictive alternative. Arrangements must provide a minimal restriction to patient's freedom and civil rights. Finally, a civil commitment must use due process. During commitment proceedings, mental patients must be accorded specific rights: the right to confront the person responsible for the commitment request, to have a hearing before a judge, and to be represented by an attorney at the hearing.

Laws governing civil commitment have changed a great deal over the past 25 years. Prior to 1969, involuntary hospitalization of mental patients in most states simply required that patients be judged "in need of treatment." This was in part the result of the view that treatment was a benevolent act and in the best interests of everyone concerned. During the '60s, many began to question US social institutions, including long-held views about the rights of people with mental disorders. In 1969, California adopted a radically different commitment standard. To be committed, an individual had to be judged dangerous to himself or others or gravely disabled. Today, most states have adopted these criteria.

Deinstitutionalization resulted in thousands of chronic mental patients being released from state hospitals across the US More than four-fifths of the involuntary (committed) psychiatric patients who lived in public psychiatric hospitals at the beginning of the 1960s have been released into the community. this has resulted in the closing of many public psychiatric hospitals and a substantial reduction in the number of hospitalized patients.

Deinstitutionalization has only been moderately successful. Today, there are too few community residences, too few community mental health centers with staff workers willing and able to care for chronic mental patients, and too few sheltered work environments. Having nowhere else to go, many individuals with mental disorders have literally ended up on the streets. Studies of homeless adults with a history of previous psychiatric hospitalization show that these individuals (a) are least likely to use emergency shelters, (b) have been homeless almost twice as long as others, (c) have a poor mental health status, (d) abuse alcohol and drugs, and (e) are involved in criminal activities.

Patients Rights

During the 1960s and 1970s, when courts were asked to consider the rights of patients committed to public psychiatric hospitals, several decisions resulted in increased patient rights. Many judges decided that even committed psychiatric patients had a right to many of the same legal safeguards the Constitution guaranteed defendants in criminal cases. Today, being either a voluntary or an involuntary patient in a mental hospital does not by itself deprive you of your civil rights. The four basic rights of all patients are:

1. Right to treatment. This right was first recognized in 1971 in the well-known Wyatt v. Stickney decision of an Alabama federal district court. Before this time, many patients who had been involuntarily committed to underfunded institutions did not receive treatment. Instead, they stayed in the institution because no one else would assume responsibility for them.

2. Right to least restrictive alternative. The Donaldson v. O'Connor decision established that people who are mentally ill cannot be confined to psychiatric hospitals for indefinite custodial periods simply because no one else can or will assume responsibility for them. At least three-quarters of the states have adopted laws based on a related suit, Youngberg v. Romeo, which affirmed that the right to the least restrictive alternative also applies to the locked wards in which committed patients were previously kept.

3. Right to refuse treatment. The history of this right dates back to 1914, when Supreme Court Justice Benjamin Cardozo stated, "Every human being of adult years and sound mind has a right to determine what shall be done with his own body, and a surgeon who performs an operation without his patient's consent commits an assault, for which he is liable for damages." In a 1978 case, Rennie v. Klein, a depressed schizophrenic patient was given the qualified right to refuse antipsychotic medication that he feared would cause him permanent harm. The judge imposed qualifications, however, that required determining (a) whether the patient would be more likely to injure himself or others if he were not medicated, (b) whether other effective treatments were available, and (c) whether the patient's belief that the medications prescribed for him were potentially dangerous was valid. A subsequent decision, Rogers v. Okin, questioned the Rennie decision given the effectiveness of the medications now given to committed psychotic patients. Many mental health professional believe that the right to refuse treatment is of questionable logic, particularly when seriously disturbed individuals refuse treatment that will actually restore their health.

4. Right to privacy. Psychiatric patients have the right to expect the professionals who care for them to respect their privacy by entering only those areas of their lives directly relevant to the clinical situation. Because it is not always possible to distinguish what is relevant in the personal history of a patient from what is not, patients and psychologists may disagree about where to draw that line. However, certain kinds of behaviors by mental health professionals that infringe on patients privacy are always out of bounds. These include unnecessarily calling patients at home or inquiring about intimate details of patients' sexual histories when they have sought treatment for different problems. Likewise, mental health professional have both socially agreed on and legal rights to privacy. For instance, patients are not supposed to try to involve themselves in their therapists' personal lives.

When applied to relationships between patients and therapists, the term confidentiality has a very specific meaning. Like those between attorneys and their clients, these are privileged relationships. Only under very special, restricted circumstances can therapists reveal the contents of conversations or other information about patients.

Competency and Responsibility

Competency to Stand Trial. The usual standard to assess competency was first stated in 1960 in Dusky v. United States, "The test must be whether he [the defendant] has sufficient present ability to consult with his lawyer with a reasonable degree of rational understanding and whether he has a rational as well as factual understanding of the proceedings against him."

The Insanity Defense. The insanity defense dates back at least to the thirteenth century. The general premise is that it is unfair to accuse someone of something that he or she cannot comprehend or to convict a person of a crime they may have not intended to commit. Over the past 150 years, four standards have guided US courts and judges in deciding criminal cases involving the insanity defense:

1, M'Naughten standard. In 1843, Daniel M'Naughten mistakenly shot at the secretary to the prime minister of England (he was trying to shoot the prime minister), but was found not guilty by reason of insanity. Public outcry resulting in a group of judges being asked to suggest a more acceptable basis for making such determinations in the future. Their recommendation that "at the time of committing of the act, the party accused was laboring under such a defect of reason, from disease of the mind, as not to know the nature and quality of the act he was doing; or if he did know it, that he did not know he was doing what was wrong."

2. Irresistible impulse standard. A major concern with the M'Naughten standard is the emphasis on cognitive factors (knowing) and corresponding deemphasis on feeling, wanting, or being able to control impulses. The irresistible impulse standard asks, "Did he know right from wrong. . . ? If he did . . ., he may nevertheless not be legally responsible if the two following conditions concur: (1) If, by reason of the duress of such mental disease, he had so far lost the power to choose between right and wrong, and to avoid doing the act in question, that his free agency was at the time destroyed; (2) and if, at the same time, the alleged crime was so connected with such mental disease, in the relation of cause and effect, as to have been the product of it."

3. Durham standard. In 1954, a broader standard of insanity defense was proposed: "An accused is not criminally responsible if his unlawful act was the product of mental disease or defect." The effect of this standard was to shift the focus of the criminal defense from whether the defendant knew the difference between right and wrong (as with the M'Naughten standard) or had lost the power to choose between right and wrong (as with the irresistible impulse standard) to a single clinical judgment: Was the crime a product of mental disorder?

4. American Law Institute (ALI) standard. The ALI standard provides the following guidelines. First, a person is not responsible for criminal conduct if at the time of such conduct he lacks substantial capacity as a result of mental disease or defect either to appreciate the criminality of his conduct or to conform his conduct to the requirements of the law. (This guideline combines the essentials of M'Naughten and Irresistible Impulse.) Second, The terms mental disease and defect do not include an abnormality manifested only by repeated criminal or otherwise antisocial conduct. (This prohibits the use of antisocial personality disorder as a defense.)

Ethical Issues

Every mental health organization has an elaborate set of ethical standards to guide its members' professional behavior. Ethical guidelines detail the association's ethical expectations of its members and discuss solutions to particularly difficult ethical problems. The states have incorporated many of these ethical guidelines into their licensing laws.

The ethical standards for psychologists has very specific guidelines about sexual involvement between the therapist and patient. Specifically, the guidelines state that "psychologists do not engage in sexual intimacies with current patients or clients." Similarly, psychologists do not take patients or clients into therapy with whom they have previously had sexual relationships and psychologists do not develop sexual relationships with former patients or clients until at least 2 years after the end of therapy. Penalties for violation of these principles are harsh, yet therapist/patient sexual involvement continues to be an issue for every mental health professional who provides clinical services. Surveys suggest that up to 12 percent of all therapists may have engaged in this behavior at least once in their professional careers.

The damage that sexual involvement between a therapist and patient causes the patient is well documented. Patient self-esteem suffers, guilt is induced, depression is intensified, and suicidal thoughts and attempts may result. These relationships almost always make future efforts at treatment more difficult.

Correctional psychologists often face ethical dilemmas created by the constant conflict in prisons between treatment concerns and security concerns. Often the psychologist is caught in conflict between the traditional role as therapist and humane advocate and role as the enforcer of custody and security.

Military psychologists are caught between the military's need to know as much as possible about its personnel (including mental status) and the psychologist's need to be able to reassure clients of the confidential nature of their relationship.

Ethical Issues in Research

Ethical issues are not confined to clinical settings. Research on AIDS provides unique problems. For example, should research staff be required to participate in AIDS work despite the minuscule possibility of their becoming infected? Can AIDS researchers guarantee confidentiality to subjects? How does one handle a situation wherein an AIDS infected individual will not share this information with past and present sexual partners?

Animal researchers must deal with the situation wherein an animal must be hurt or killed as part of the research. Psychotherapy research often uses control groups wherein some participants are given a placebo treatment. Researchers studying special populations are often not as familiar with the specialized literature on these groups. As a result, researchers may conclude that their findings were influenced by subjects' age or sex when an adequate grasp of the research literature would have lead them to a different conclusion.

Ethical Standards and the Law

A recent report of the Ethics Committee of the American Psychological Association summarized the ethical violations it investigated during 1991 and 1992. The most common investigation was for inappropriate professional practice, followed by dual relationships, inappropriate teaching, research or administration, and inappropriate advertising and public statements. The number of ethics cases brought to the Ethics Committee of APA continues to climb.

KEY IDEAS AND OBJECTIVES FOR STUDENTS

After reading the chapter, you should be able to answer each of the following questions:

1. On what issues must mental health professionals render expert judgments? What is the Tarasoff standard?

2. For whom is civil commitment indicated and what are the limits on its use?

3. What are the four specific rights of patients? What standards have resulted from deciding the insanity defense?

4. What are the ethical standards for professional behavior for psychology and to whom do they apply?

Legal and Ethical Issues in the Movies

1. Final Analysis (1992, Warner Home Video, 124 min). This film provides insights into ethical dilemmas when Richard Gere, who plays a psychiatrist, decides to have an affair with a patient's attractive sister. Many of the situations in the film border on the preposterous and do not always provide the most appropriate model for dealing with ethical dilemmas.

2. Nuts (1987, Warner Home Video, 118 min). Barbara Streisand plays an eccentric prostitute trying to prove that she is mentally fit to stand trial. The film is an excellent example of the issues involved in the assessment of insanity and competence to stand trial.

Questions after watching the movies.

Final Analysis

1. Why are sexual relationships with clients (or family members of clients) problematic? What were some of the "poor" decisions made by Richard Gere's character?

2. How could the film have better dealt with the ethical issues?

Nuts

1. Which of the insanity standards discussed in the text were referred to in the film? Did the film present these issues in an appropriate manner? What were the major consistencies (or inconsistencies) with the material found in the text?

2. What new ideas were presented in the film about the issue of competence to stand trial and insanity? If you were asked to serve as an expert witness, what decision would you have made regarding Barbara Streisand's character?

Using Case Studies in Abnormal Behavior by Meyer and Osborne: Legal Issues

General Summary

Chapter 16 provides a useful table showing the "Taxonomy of Psycholegal Issues" including both criminal and civil issues. Three cases are presented which focus on (a) legal competence, (b) malingering, and (c) criminal responsibility and dangerousness.

Case Comparisons

Central Nervous System Dysfunction and Legal Incompetence due to Aging and/or Alcohol: The Case of Ingrid. In this case, the client began to drink heavily following the death of her spouse. Her son petitioned to have her mother legally incompetent. The court agreed initially with the son, but it was later overturned. What factors led to the initial decision? Why was it overturned? Was an error made initially or were other factors related?

Malingering, Factitious Disorder, or True Disorder: The Case of the Wound that Never Heals. This case illustrates the problem with diagnosis of malingering. What factors lead to a belief that this patient was malingering? How was the diagnosis factitious disorder made? What are the consequences of an incorrect diagnosis?

Criminal Responsibility, Competency to Stand Trial, and Dangerousness: The Case of John Hinckley. John Hinckley was found not guilty by reason of insanity for the 1981 assassination attempt on President Ronald Regan. This decision resulted in 26 different bills introduced into legislation to modify the federal statute that covers the insanity defense. Given what you have read about these legal issues, was the court decision correct? Should the laws be changes? Why? Why not?

Integrating Perspectives
A Biopsychosocial Model

The Case of Ingrid:

Biological Factors

- Ingrid began to drink heavily and alcohol has significant effects on brain functioning.

Psychological Factors

- Loss of a spouse can play a role in the decision to drink as well as bring on depression that may have influenced her cognitive functioning.
- All indications are that Ingrid had few if any psychological problems before the loss of her husband. This likely served as a buffer to help her recover so quickly.

Social Factors

- In the short term, loss of a life-long companion was overwhelming. However, she was able to eventually learn to cope with the loss. Her son's concern over loosing his inheritance may have contributed to his overreacting to the situation.

Sample Multiple-Choice Questions

1. The ________________ requires that therapists do whatever they can to warn persons threatened during the course of psychotherapy.
   a. APA Ethical Code
   b. Tarasoff Standard
   c. Durham Standard
   d. M'Naughten Code

2. You receive a phone call from Dr. Skaar, a psychologist at the university clinic. Dr. Skaar explains to you that she has been seeing a client who is infatuated with Debbie, the woman you have been dating for 6 months. Dr. Skaar's client has indicated that he has considered killing you to end your relationship with Debbie. Dr. Skaar has reported her concerns to the police, and is calling you since it is her duty to warn you that you are in danger. What standard is Dr. Skaar following?
   a. Poddar Standard
   b. Tarasoff Standard
   c. Durham Standard
   d. M'Naughten Standard

3. Dr. Long is a professor at a large northeastern university who was being seen at the university counseling center. He has a great deal of difficulty controlling his anger and frequently screams at his colleagues and students when they don't agree with him. He actually punched out a student who disagreed with a grade that he received in an introductory course. Therapy has focused on these issues, but he has not made much progress. He was recently denied tenure and told his therapist that he plans to kill the chair of his department. Based on research for risk of violence, is Dr. Long at risk for following through with his threats? why?
   a. Yes, men are more likely to harm others than women.
   b. Yes, anger control may be predictive of individuals who commit violent acts.
   c. No, professors are rarely involved in violent acts.
   d. No, individuals who are seeking counseling rarely commit violent acts.

4. People must be judged ________________ to be psychiatrically committed.
   a. unable to care for their own needs
   b. mentally ill but not necessarily dangerous
   c. dangerous but not necessarily mentally ill
   d. mentally ill and dangerous

5. Judy's father was committed to a mental hospital in 1954 after he was diagnosed with schizophrenia. Judy was recently evaluated at the university medical center and she received the same diagnosis. What is the likelihood that Judy will also be committed to a mental hospital against her wishes.
   a. Low, prior to 1960, proof of mental illness was sufficient for an involuntary commitment, but not today.
   b. Low, schizophrenia is easily treated today and Judy will be cured before she leave the hospital.
   c. High, familial schizophrenia typically results in excessive violence, thus Judy will likely require total hospitalization.
   d. High, today, the diagnosis of mental illness is grounds for involuntary commitment.

6. The number of patients hospitalized in psychiatric facilities peaked in _______.
   a. the late 1890s.
   b. the early 1920s.
   c. the late 1930s.
   d. the early 1950s.

7. Deinstitutionalization is seen by many to have failed because _________.
   a. mental patients do better in hospital settings
   b. states failed to plan and pay for community treatment programs
   c. there were too few psychologists working in the community
   d. all of these factors have contributed to the failure of deinstitutionalization.

8. Bachrach's study on the homeless focused on the special problems of mentally ill women. These women are likely to be
   a. sexually exploited
   b. stigmatized for their mental disorders.
   c. involved in crime.
   d. all of the above.

9. The purpose of ethical guidelines is to _________________.
   a. protect the profession from unnecessary lawsuits.
   b. provide detailed information about ethical expectations.
   c. make it more likely that members will engage in ethical behavior.
   d. provide information about legal issues related to the practice of psychology.

10. In 1992 the American Psychological Association found that ________ percent of the professionals were involved in inappropriate professional practices.
   a. 11
   b. 32
   c. 54
   d. 87

Answer Key

1. b
2. b
3. b
4. d
5. a
6. d
7. b
8. d
9. c
10. b